SLEEP – PHYSIOLOGY, FUNCTIONS, DREAMING AND DISORDERS

CHILDREN AND SLEEP

MANAGEMENT, HEALTH EFFECTS AND GENDER DIFFERENCES

SLEEP – PHYSIOLOGY, FUNCTIONS, DREAMING AND DISORDERS

Additional books and e-books in this series can be found on Nova's website under the Series tab.

SLEEP – PHYSIOLOGY, FUNCTIONS, DREAMING AND DISORDERS

CHILDREN AND SLEEP

MANAGEMENT, HEALTH EFFECTS AND GENDER DIFFERENCES

OLIVIE GADBOIS
EDITOR

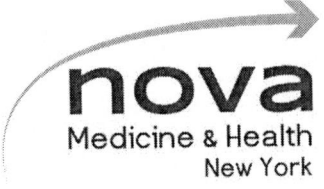

Copyright © 2020 by Nova Science Publishers, Inc.

All rights reserved. No part of this book may be reproduced, stored in a retrieval system or transmitted in any form or by any means: electronic, electrostatic, magnetic, tape, mechanical photocopying, recording or otherwise without the written permission of the Publisher.

We have partnered with Copyright Clearance Center to make it easy for you to obtain permissions to reuse content from this publication. Simply navigate to this publication's page on Nova's website and locate the "Get Permission" button below the title description. This button is linked directly to the title's permission page on copyright.com. Alternatively, you can visit copyright.com and search by title, ISBN, or ISSN.

For further questions about using the service on copyright.com, please contact:
Copyright Clearance Center
Phone: +1-(978) 750-8400   Fax: +1-(978) 750-4470   E-mail: info@copyright.com

NOTICE TO THE READER

The Publisher has taken reasonable care in the preparation of this book, but makes no expressed or implied warranty of any kind and assumes no responsibility for any errors or omissions. No liability is assumed for incidental or consequential damages in connection with or arising out of information contained in this book. The Publisher shall not be liable for any special, consequential, or exemplary damages resulting, in whole or in part, from the readers' use of, or reliance upon, this material. Any parts of this book based on government reports are so indicated and copyright is claimed for those parts to the extent applicable to compilations of such works.

Independent verification should be sought for any data, advice or recommendations contained in this book. In addition, no responsibility is assumed by the Publisher for any injury and/or damage to persons or property arising from any methods, products, instructions, ideas or otherwise contained in this publication.

This publication is designed to provide accurate and authoritative information with regard to the subject matter covered herein. It is sold with the clear understanding that the Publisher is not engaged in rendering legal or any other professional services. If legal or any other expert assistance is required, the services of a competent person should be sought. FROM A DECLARATION OF PARTICIPANTS JOINTLY ADOPTED BY A COMMITTEE OF THE AMERICAN BAR ASSOCIATION AND A COMMITTEE OF PUBLISHERS.

Additional color graphics may be available in the e-book version of this book.

Library of Congress Cataloging-in-Publication Data

ISBN: 978-1-53618-074-9

Published by Nova Science Publishers, Inc. † New York

CONTENTS

Preface		vii
Chapter 1	Clinical Assessment of Pediatric Sleep Disorders *Mollie E. Rischard, Devin R. Barlaan and Lisa D. Cromer*	1
Chapter 2	Sleep Disorders in Pediatric Populations: Clinical Features, Etiologies, Comorbidities, and Rule-Outs *Mollie E. Rischard, Devin R. Barlaan and Lisa D. Cromer*	31
Chapter 3	The Importance of Sleep on Childhood Neurodevelopment *Negin Badihian and Roya Kelishadi*	79
Chapter 4	Emotional and Behavioral Disturbances and Sleep Problems in Children *Igor A. Kelmanson*	99

Chapter 5	From Mouth Breathing to Pediatric Obstructive Sleep Apnea: Consequences, Diagnosis and Treatment Options	115
	Maria Christina Thomé Pacheco, Fabiana Vasconcelos Campos and Maria Teresa Martins de Araújo	

Index   **169**

Preface

Children and Sleep: Management, Health Effects and Gender Differences begins by delineating the measurement tools currently available to evaluate sleep problems in children and adolescents: polysomnography, actigraphy, sleep diaries, and questionnaires.

Continuing, this collection unpacks the complexities of the most common sleep disorders affecting children and adolescents by discussing the child-specific features, etiology, common comorbidities, and differential diagnostic considerations pertinent for each disorder.

The authors summarize the importance of a healthy sleep cycle in normal brain development during childhood and the effects of sleep disturbances on normal brain function and brain structure.

Additionally, possible associations between sleep disturbances in children and emotional/behavioral problems are addressed, based on a suggestion that these symptoms are not the emerging manifestations of an underlying disorder but rather are a network of symptoms that are causally interrelated.

In closing, the authors highlight the importance of identifying the causes of mouth breathing and obstructive sleep apnea in children. If left untreated, such breathing disorders can progress to more severe conditions in adulthood.

Chapter 1 - The evolution and expansion of pediatric sleep science has led to an increased demand for reliable and valid measurement tools. Today there are both objective and subjective tools available to evaluate varying pediatric sleep concerns. These measurement methods are extensive and can be challenging for healthcare providers to navigate. The purpose of this chapter is to delineate the measurement tools currently available to evaluate sleep problems in children and adolescents: polysomnography, actigraphy, sleep diaries, and questionnaires. The authors describe each assessment method and its respective clinical indications; they then review costs, discuss strengths and weaknesses of each approach, and address child-related considerations for administering the measures. The chapter concludes by summarizing the findings and offering recommendations for future research.

Chapter 2 - Pediatric sleep disorders are varied and complex, which can impede accurate detection. The present chapter reviews the most common sleep disorders affecting children and adolescents. Specifically, this chapter unpacks the complexities of these pathologies by discussing the child-specific features, etiology, common comorbidities, and differential diagnostic considerations pertinent for each disorder.

Chapter 3 - Sleep is an essential time and process in human life. We spend almost one third of our life sleeping or trying to fall asleep. It is especially important when it comes to minors; about forty percent of the childhood period is spent in sleep. Intense brain activities that involve higher cortical functions and significant physiological activities occur during sleep. Therefore, it led some scientists to conclude that brain is more active during sleep compared to the wakeful state. Sleep is considered to have influential roles in neural plasticity, brain development, and skill learning during childhood. Moreover, it would affect capability of acquiring new skills and exploring the environment when facing a new situation. It is reported that one third of children experience some degrees of sleep disturbances. The circadian and homeostatic systems are both responsible for sleep regulation. Sleep duration, quality, timing, regularity, and absence of sleep disturbances are all important for the proper function of brain and body. The adequate duration of sleep varies between individuals; it is influenced by the complex interactions of genetic and environmental factors. But in general, the required duration of sleep is much longer in newborns, i.e., 12-16 hours a day, and has a gradual decrease to 8-10 hours a day in teenagers. The proportion of rapid eye movement (REM) and non-REM sleeps are also affected by age because of the different functions of these states. While newborns have equal REM and non-REM duration, REM sleep would gradually decrease as the child grows up. Sleep problems diminish normal brain function and would result in short- and long-term adverse health effects. Inadequate sleep duration or quality during childhood might cause dysfunctions in the attention, behavior, cognition, and working memory, which in turn would cause hyperactivity and poor impulse control, decreased intellectual ability, and learning problems. It would further increase the risk of hypertension, obesity, diabetes, and other psychological problems including depression. However, increased duration of daily sleep would also result in hypertension, diabetes, obesity and psychological disorders. Additionally, sleep disturbances can affect high level cognitive functions (e.g., abstract thinking and cognitive flexibility) and even might affect brain morphology in distinct regions. In this chapter, the authors aim to summarize the importance of healthy sleep cycle in normal brain development during childhood and the effects of sleep disturbances on normal brain function and brain structure.

Chapter 4 - Disturbed sleep is commonly reported among typically developing children, and the term 'sleep-related problems' is commonly used in research in this field and can encompass a variety of issues. In cross-sectional epidemiological studies, sleep disturbances are reported in 25–45% of school-aged children. Bedtime resistance, sleep related anxiety, sleep initiation problems, insufficient hours of sleep, night waking and daytime fatigue and tiredness are sleep problems frequently reported in school aged children. The types of reported sleep problems vary with age.

An important, although insufficiently addressed issue, is possible association between sleep problems and the signs of emotional/behavioral disturbances in children. Several studies have explored the association between sleep problems and combined anxiety/depression symptomatology. Sleep problems are not currently part of the diagnostic criteria of externalizing disorders, but have been linked to aggression, attention problems, and substance use in youth. Little is currently known about associations among sleep problems and oppositional defiant disorder, although this disorder is at the intersection of internalizing and externalizing disorders and also tends to precede depression and generalized anxiety disorder.

This paper addresses possible associations between sleep disturbances in children and emotional/behavioral problems with a new look at their co-occurrences based on a suggestion that these symptoms and signs are not the emerging manifestations of an underlying disorder but rather are a network of symptoms, dynamic complex system or dynamic constellation of symptoms (and signs) that are causally interrelated.

Chapter 5 - Pediatric obstructive sleep apnea (OSA) is – much like in the adult form of the disease – caused by the abnormal blockage of the upper airway during sleep. As a rather pliant conduit, the upper airway is naturally subject to collapsing, becoming even more so during sleep and when extrinsic factors, such as craniofacial alterations and breathing disorders, are in place.

The shaping of the palate and upper airway structures begins with the sucking and swallowing that take place *in utero*. At birth and during early childhood, the coordination between sucking, swallowing, chewing and nasal breathing plays a significant role in the development of the human face, affecting the expansion of craniofacial structures and the shape taken by the upper airway.

Breathing disorders involving obstruction of the upper airway are often the reason why children breathe through their mouths. The persistence of mouth breathing throughout the development compromises facial bones and the positioning of teeth, affecting the stomatognathic system and even the body's posture. Thus, if a child does not breathe properly, she cannot swallow, chew or talk so.

The younger the child at the onset of such sleep-related breathing disorders, the more severe the outcome later in life. Therefore, an early diagnosis of pediatric OSA through the identification of potential risk factors could, at the very least, decrease the impact this particular disorder has over the lives of afflicted subjects. It is, however, rather more complicated to diagnose OSA in children than in the adult population, save in cases when the symptoms are particularly severe. An integrated, multidisciplinary approach is, therefore, necessary not only to diagnose but also to treat the pediatric form of this disease.

This chapter addresses the details on how the replacement of nasal breathing by mouth breathing in childhood affects the development of facial structures and the upper airway, compromising the dental arches and making children more vulnerable to OSA.

The authors will discuss the consequences of persistent mouth breathing and upper airway obstructions, as well as of deleterious oral habits and the very body posture adopted by the child. The authors shall then focus on the main causes underlying sleep-disordered breathing, along with a detailed review on clinical procedures and complementary exams that, combined with the indispensable polysomnography with capnography, assist in the difficult diagnosis of OSA in children. Finally, the authors will conduct a thorough discussion on treatment options available for such patients.

With this chapter, the authors endeavor to highlight the importance of identifying the causes behind the development of mouth breathing and OSA in children, for, if left untreated, such breathing disorders can progress to more severe conditions in adulthood.

In: Children and Sleep
Editor: Olivie Gadbois

ISBN: 978-1-53618-074-9
© 2020 Nova Science Publishers, Inc.

Chapter 1

CLINICAL ASSESSMENT OF PEDIATRIC SLEEP DISORDERS

Mollie E. Rischard[*], *Devin R. Barlaan* *and Lisa D. Cromer, PhD*
Department of Psychology,
The University of Tulsa, Tulsa, OK, US

ABSTRACT

The evolution and expansion of pediatric sleep science has led to an increased demand for reliable and valid measurement tools. Today there are both objective and subjective tools available to evaluate varying pediatric sleep concerns. These measurement methods are extensive and can be challenging for healthcare providers to navigate. The purpose of this chapter is to delineate the measurement tools currently available to evaluate sleep problems in children and adolescents: polysomnography, actigraphy, sleep diaries, and questionnaires. We describe each assessment method and its respective clinical indications; we then review costs, discuss strengths and weaknesses of each approach, and address child-related considerations for administering the measures. The chapter

---

[*] Corresponding Author's Email: mer597@utulsa.edu.

concludes by summarizing the findings and offering recommendations for future research.

CLINICAL ASSESSMENT OF PEDIATRIC SLEEP DISORDERS

The measurement of pediatric sleep problems has burgeoned since the 1970s when sleep questions were first embedded in daytime psychopathology screening tools, such as Achenbach's Child Behavioral Checklist (CBCL; Achenbach, 1991) and Conner's Ratings scales (Conner, 1970). Sleep problems being incorporated into screening tools reflected the science at the time: there was a general understanding that sleep and mental health were related. Sleep-specific questionnaires emerged in the 1980s as pediatric sleep became a field of study in its own right (Bruni et al., 1996). Today, there are numerous objective and subjective sleep tools for the practitioner to navigate. This chapter reviews the most common methods: polysomnography, actigraphy, sleep diaries, and questionnaires. The chapter explains each instrument and what it is most useful in assessing; we then review costs, discuss strengths and weaknesses of each approach, and address child-related considerations for administering the measures. We conclude the chapter by summarizing the findings and offering recommendations for future research.

POLYSOMNOGRAPHY

Polysomnography and actigraphy are objective methods of sleep assessment. Polysomnography (PSG) is a diagnostic, and records biophysiological parameters continuously and simultaneously across a sleep period. Commonly referred to as a sleep study, PSG is typically conducted by a sleep technologist and most often occurs in a sleep lab within a sleep disorders unit at a hospital or sleep center (American Sleep Disorders Association [ASDA], 1997). In this setting, the patient is observed overnight for at least one night. PSG can also be administered in a person's home. For at-home administration, a sleep technologist sets up the necessary equipment in the child's home and includes an audio-visual recording device because the technologist does not stay overnight (Brockmann et al., 2013). Regarding setup for both in-home and laboratory PSG, the sleep technologist places electrodes on the child's scalp, chin, chest, and legs using adhesive tape (Beck & Marcus, 2009). These electrodes record several physiological parameters, described below (ASDA, 1997).

PSG documents sleep stages, which are identified by changes in brain waves, eye movements, and muscle tone. Other physiological parameters measured by PSG include respiratory function, which comprises air flow at the nose and mouth, respiratory movements of the chest and abdomen, a pulse indicator, limb movements, electrical activity of the heart, and sounds such as snoring or other vocalizations (Wise & Glaze, 2019). Scoring and interpretation of all physiological measures collected are based on standardized scoring that has been published by the American Academy of Sleep Medicine (Iber & Iber, 2007).

Scoring and interpreting a sleep study is a multi-step process. First, the entire sleep study is divided into 30-second "epochs," for the review to be conducted (American Academy of Sleep Medicine [AASM], 2007). For example, if a pediatric patient slept 10 hours (or 600 minutes), 1200 epochs would be identified. Then, the epochs are reviewed by the sleep technologist three times. During the first review, the technologist identifies the sleep stages and arousals using EEG data (AASM, 2007). The second review examines respiratory events in order to determine the presence of apneas or hypopneas, which involve the absence or reduction of air flow respectively. The third pass scores limb movements and abnormalities in cardiac function (AASM, 2007). The sleep technologist generates a report by synthesizing and scoring the various sleep parameters (AASM, 2007). Following the sleep technologist's scoring, a sleep physician interprets the entire sleep study with respect to the three sleep parameters: a) sleep stages and arousals, b) respiratory events, and c) limb movements and cardiac activity (AASM, 2007). Altogether, scoring, interpreting, and communicating the findings through the written report can take approximately 6 to 7 hours of effort (AASM, 2007).

Clinical Indications

PSG is the only way to diagnose obstructive sleep apnea, narcolepsy, periodic limb movement disorder, and nocturnal seizures (Aurora et al., 2012; Beck & Marcus, 2009). PSG is not typically indicated for common pediatric sleep pathologies such as parasomnias, insomnia, or restless legs syndrome that can easily be detected via less expensive and less invasive means, such as a sleep diary or sleep history assessment (Beck & Marcus, 2009). However, a sleep study might be a necessary step in order to determine a pathological cause for common pediatric sleep problems like bedtime resistance, night awakenings, or excessive daytime sleepiness (Beck & Marcus, 2009). For example, if a child suffers from nighttime arousals, and a clinician is unsure if these are environmentally caused or are biologically driven, PSG might be indicated in order to identify if a child's sudden night arousals are caused by disordered breathing. Similarly, if a child has long standing delays in sleep onset which may be behaviorally driven but also could be due to a medical issue, PSG would provide definitive evidence as to whether delayed sleep onset was the result of restless legs syndrome, insomnia, or a parasomnia like nightmare disorder.

Costs

PSG costs vary based on setting of in-home or lab. A recent review estimated in-home testing to be approximately $400 a night and lab testing to be approximately $700 a night (Stewart et al., 2017). Although in-home PSG is more cost effective, this review indicated higher rates of false negatives with in-home testing, meaning that in-home tests may not detect disorders that are actually present (Stewart et al., 2017). An additional cost consideration is that insurance companies may only cover costs when the test verifies a medical need. In other words, negative tests could require patients to pay out-of-pocket (Stewart et al., 2017), therefore PSG may not be utilized for rule-out considerations or for mild to moderate cases of sleep disorders.

Strengths and Limitations

Because PSG comprehensively and objectively measures a significant number of biophysiological markers, it is considered the gold standard for objective sleep assessment in pediatric populations (Marcus, 2001). The standardized scoring criteria (Iber & Iber, 2007) affords a high level of reliability and validity in diagnostic decision making, allowing for seamless comparison of results across research laboratories.

PSG has several limitations. First, individuals undergoing laboratory PSG assessment must adapt to the unfamiliar and restrictive laboratory environment (Katz et al., 2002). Adjusting to a novel environment is challenging by itself, but managing the additional potential disturbances unique to PSG - such as the electrodes on the body, limited mobility caused by the wires and cables, and the pressure of being observed while sleeping – can substantially hinder the quality and quantity of sleep (Newell et al., 2012). While the novel setting is not an issue for in-home PSG, the invasive setup can still interfere markedly with a person's sleep. These impediments can cause a first night-effect (Agnew et al., 1966) for patients (Newell et al., 2012; Scholle et al., 2003). The first-night effect is associated with diminished sleep quality including more wake time, less REM sleep, and increased REM and stage 4 latencies in the first night of a sleep study. Therefore, the first-night effect can significantly disrupt the sleep architecture which can render the assessment on the first night invalid. When this occurs, the patient typically needs to be studied during a second night of sleep in order for this effect to attenuate (Agnew et al., 1966). Data concerning the first-night effect has led researchers to conclude that a single night of PSG is insufficient in most cases and results in questionable diagnostic accuracy, in particular, higher rates of type I error (Newell et al., 2012).

Child Considerations

PSG presents unique challenges in pediatric populations (Beck & Marcus, 2009). From a child's point of view, sleeping overnight in an unfamiliar environment with multiple physiologic sensors attached to their body can feel frightening and invasive, provoking fear and anxiety (Zaremba et al., 2005). PSG technologists report that young children can be uncooperative making setup and connectivity with instrumentation difficult (Beck & Marcus, 2009; Zaremba et al., 2005). Poor or inconsistent connectivity can interfere with electrode placement and signal integrity, thus compromising the validity of the assessment (Zaremba et al., 2005). Additionally, if parents are distressed seeing their child attached to medical equipment, they may be less effective at comforting an anxious child (Zaremba et al., 2005).

In order to minimize and manage these unique challenges for administering PSG with children, pediatric sleep centers can try to create a child-friendly and family-oriented environment (Beck & Marcus, 2010; Zaremba et al., 2005). A child-focused model might include psychological preparation for the child, providing a developmentally appropriate sleeping space, and modifying staffing and lab hours to accommodate earlier bedtimes for children (Beck & Marcus, 2010; Zaremba et al., 2005). Technicians may be trained to be mindful of parental anxiety throughout the PSG process, and work to also put the parent at-ease. Therefore, orientation to the testing procedures involves both the parent as well as the child, and both parent and child are allowed to have all questions answered before and during the testing (Beck & Marcus, 2009). Also, parents may be allowed to spend the night with their child during the assessment.

ACTIGRAPHY

Actigraphy is an unobtrusive, computerized wristwatch-like device that objectively measures sleep patterns. Actigraphy is widely used because it is small, uncomplicated, and can be worn continuously with minimal disruption for the wearer (Galland et al., 2018). Unlike PSG, actigraphy does not directly measure sleep-wake patterns; rather, the device infers sleep and wake patterns based on the absence or presence of movement and by detecting light (Ancoli-Israel et al., 2003; Galland et al., 2018). Many actigraphy devices contain accelerometer-based motion sensors, which record activity counts across defined epochs (Galland et al., 2018). Epoch lengths vary across devices; in pediatric populations, epochs are commonly reported in 60-second intervals (Meltzer et al., 2012). Actigraphy scoring algorithms define each epoch of recorded activity as either sleep or wake by weighting the activity scores of the surrounding minutes. This data is extracted via computer-based software systems interfacing with the actigraphy device (Meltzer et al., 2012).

There is currently no standard procedure for recording key actigraphy-derived sleep parameters, such as sleep onset/offset or nocturnal wake frequency as well as scoring the recorded actigraphy signals (Meltzer & Westin, 2011; Meltzer et al., 2012). Manuals that accompany actigraphy devices provide some guidance on how to manually set scoring intervals (Meltzer & Westin, 2011), but for the most part, researchers recommend using scoring rules reported in methods sections of published studies in order to determine interval start and stop times (e.g., Acebo & LeBourgeios, 2006). Unfortunately, this recommendation is challenging to comply with when scoring rules are inconsistently reported across actigraphy studies (Meltzer & Westin, 2011). Researchers have called for the development of standard actigraphy-based scoring procedures in order to address this issue (Meltzer & Westin, 2011).

When interpreting results, it is important to consider actigraphy's sensitivity, or accuracy, in identifying sleep periods, and specificity, or precision, in detecting wakefulness. A systematic review conducted by Meltzer and colleagues (2012) examined actigraphy's true positive rates and true negative rates across 10 validation-like studies from a cumulative sample of 931 children. Although these studies utilized different devices, recording parameters, and scoring algorithms, they uniformly reported high levels of sensitivity readings of sleep periods, with indices ranging from 88.2 to 99.3 (Meltzer et al., 2012). That is, across studies, actigraphy was consistently good at identifying sleep periods (Meltzer et al., 2012). When examining specificity, for measuring wakefulness among pediatric populations, the researchers found that among the 10 validation-like studies, 55% of the specificities reported were less than 60.0, with values ranging from 24.0 to 76.9 (Meltzer et al., 2012). In other words, actigraphy under-identified wakefulness, in that over half of the studies found that actigraphy correctly defined wakefulness less than 60% of the time. These findings suggest that actigraphy might over-estimate children's total sleep time. Because actigraphy functions by detecting motion, if a child or adolescent is awake in bed, but not moving, the actigraphy device might mis-define them as sleeping. For this reason, protocols typically require caregivers to complete concurrent sleep diaries when actigraphy is used (Galland et al., 2014).

Clinical Indications

Actigraphy devices differ in quality and level of reliability and validity. Researchers and clinicians need to research which devices are suitable for assessing habitual sleep-wake cycles as well as sleep quality and maintenance (Martin & Hakim, 2011). In a clinical context, high quality actigraphy can be useful in the diagnosis of circadian-rhythm disorders, insomnia and hypersomnia, and non-REM sleep arousal disorders. Actigraphy is also frequently used to index treatment response in children with sleep disorders and behavioral problems or behavioral disorders that interfere with sleep, such as attention-deficit hyperactivity disorder (Martin & Hakim, 2011). Prior to using actigraphy for tracking change, we recommend that the clinician or researcher collect 5 to 7 days of baseline data in order to determine what is typical for a given patient on a particular actigraphy device.

Costs

The cost of actigraphy varies based on design and function. Basic devices that monitor activity and heartrate can be purchased for as little as $30. While affordable, these devices are not used in clinical research and have not been validated. More sophisticated and complex devices, that provide comprehensive, high quality data in real-time, can cost up to $300 (Stone & Ancoli-Israel, 2011).

Strengths and Limitations

There are multiple advantages of using actigraphy to understand abnormal sleep patterns (Martin & Hakim, 2011). When it comes to objective assessment, actigraphy is considered both convenient and cost-effective (Martin & Hakim, 2011). Unlike PSG, children are less likely to fear the device, and moreover, some enjoy having the special watch to wear. Actigraphy is more affordable than PSG (Stone & Ancoli-Israel, 2011) and is unobtrusive (Martin & Hakim, 2011), which all together makes these devices a feasible option for pediatric use.

Shortcomings of actigraphy assessment stem from its absence of standard scoring procedures and poor specificity. The lack of universal scoring guidelines makes it challenging to compare results across studies in order to develop normative values for key sleep variables. From a clinical perspective, lack of standard scoring criteria precludes uniformity and empirically supported clinical decision-making, which has consequences for treatment. Actigraphy's questionable specificity also poses problems. In order to obtain accurate sleep onset and offset times and cross-validate night-time arousals, sleep diaries are generally recommended as accompanying data with actigraphy assessment (Galland et al., 2014). Unfortunately, parental and individual compliance with sleep diaries are often a concern within pediatric sleep research (Galland et al., 2014). Moreover, researchers recommend wearing actigraphy devices for at least 7 consecutive days in order to obtain five nights of reliable data. Thus, families may experience burden having to also adhere to 7 consecutive days of sleep diary recordings (Galland et al., 2014).

Requiring sleep diary completion in conjunction with wearing the actigraphy device also weakens the utility of actigraphy as a single diagnostic instrument. Actigraphy is not traditionally used in isolation to make diagnostic decisions (Galland et al., 2014). Rather, the devices are typically incorporated as supplementary tools in diagnostic decision making for certain disorders and to monitor treatment progress (Galland et al., 2014). While tracking treatment response is a necessary practice in clinical care, not being able to apply the technologies as preliminary and unitary indicators of sleep pathology limits actigraphy's function as a convenient and accessible assessment tool in pediatric sleep medicine.

Child Considerations

Logistical factors can limit the utility of actigraphy for pediatric sleep assessment. First, depending on age and maturity, children might be more susceptible to losing the actigraphy watches, which can augment cost. Additionally, children might forget to regularly charge the devices, which can result in disrupted readings during the night if the device loses battery. For devices that sync with software that is specific to a laboratory computer, there is additional burden of visits for families to bring the watch in for data downloads or for lab personnel to collect the devices.

Practitioners utilizing actigraphy within pediatric populations should also consider several child-specific adaptations in order to make the assessment successful. First, practitioners should ensure that pediatric patients wear the device in such a way to maximize reliable readings and prevent misplacement. Actigraphy placement for pediatric populations is most commonly recommended on the non-dominant wrist for older children and on the ankle or calf for infants and toddlers (Sadeh & Acebo, 2002). Wrist bands should be small enough for little wrists, and clinicians and researchers should consider the size of the actigraphy watch face when ordering for young children, as some actigraphy watches may be wider than a child's wrist. To prevent the devices from losing battery life, families can set alarms as cues to charge the devices. Families can also use alarms to help them comply with concurrent daily sleep diary completion.

SLEEP DIARIES

The most commonly used subjective sleep measurement tool is the sleep diary. Recorded at home daily, using paper and pencil or recently, smartphone applications, commonly recorded sleep parameters include: sleep onset, sleep onset latency, feeling of wakefulness after initial sleep onset, presence of nightmares, total sleep time, total time in bed, and daytime sleepiness (Sadeh, 2015). These parameters are typically recorded across several nights.

For sleep diary assessment, parental report is usually preferred over child self-report in both research and clinical care (Spruyt & Gozal, 2011b), yet, studies have suggested that parents are not reliable reporters when it comes to key sleep parameters (Dayyat et al., 2011; Werner et al., 2008). Several studies have compared parental report via diary to actigraphy in order to determine parental accuracy in reporting key sleep metrics for their children. By and large, these studies have found that parents are unaware of children's night awakenings (Werner et al., 2008) and that parents tend to over-estimate total sleep time (Dayyat et al., 2011; Werner et al., 2008). Researchers have also examined agreement between caregiver and child-self report on sleep diaries. One study found that caregivers reported an idealized version of adolescent sleep, estimating substantially earlier bedtimes on school nights and weekends, significantly later wake times on weekends, and significantly more total sleep time than both adolescents self-reported and actigraphy reflected (Short et al., 2013). In order to overcome the limitation of poor parental reporting, researchers recommend allowing adolescents to complete the sleep diaries when under investigation (Short et al., 2013) as well as augmenting sleep diaries with actigraphy assessment (Werner et al., 2008).

Sleep diaries do not have a standardized format and dozens of diaries are published and widely available for use (Carney et al., 2012). Diaries vary in purpose and response structure, with some diaries utilizing Likert ratings or visual analogue scales while others use free-response formats (Carney et al., 2012). Number of questions and sleep parameters that are queried also vary widely. Because formats vary, scoring and interpretation does as well.

Lack of uniformity in diaries results in sleep metrics varying across labs and clinics. Meta-analyses for insomnia treatment studies have primarily relied upon sleep diary data to estimate treatment effect sizes (Irwin et al., 2006; Morin et al., 1994; Smith et al., 2002). However, these effect size estimates were derived from data on a variety of sleep diaries with distinctive response formats and inconsistent definitions of target sleep variables. Thus, the conclusions drawn from these and similar studies must be interpreted cautiously. Researchers have called for development of a consensus-driven, standardized sleep diary to address this concern (Carney et al., 2012).

Sleep diaries have evidenced promising psychometric properties for certain sleep variables (Rogers et al., 1993; Short et al., 2017; Werner et al., 2008). In a sample of 50 kindergarten-aged children, parental report of sleep onset, sleep offset, and assumed sleep time via sleep diary over a 7-day period showed satisfactory rates of agreement with actigraphy data (Werner et al., 2008). These findings suggest that sleep diaries are a valid index of children's sleep schedule times (Werner et al., 2008). In another study, Short and colleagues (2017) investigated how many nights of sleep diary recordings are needed for reliable estimates of sleep outcomes in a cross-national sample of 1,766 adolescent youth. The researchers examined test-retest reliability statistics for 12 days of self-report sleep diary recordings and found that intraclass correlation coefficients for bedtime, sleep onset latency, and sleep duration indicated good-to-excellent reliability from 5 weekday nights of sleep diary entries (Short et al., 2017). Thus, sleep diaries represent a reliable assessment tool for evaluating important sleep parameters in adolescent populations.

Clinical Indications

Sleep diaries are regarded as the gold standard for subjective sleep assessment (Buysse et al., 2006). Subjective sleep assessment is utilized for diagnosing insomnia, parasomnias, and delayed sleep-wake phase disorder (Sadeh, 2015). Sleep diaries can also provide augmentative information to assist in identifying disorders of hypersomnolence, restless legs syndrome, and sleep apnea. Researchers and clinicians have most commonly used sleep diaries to track intervention effects, in other words, to detect changes in sleep parameters for individual subjects or patients (Sadeh, 2015).

Costs

Sleep diaries are usually free. There are several sleep diary templates available online that can be downloaded at no cost (e.g., National Sleep Foundation's Sleep Diary). Recently, sleep diary applications have become available for download on smartphones and or tablets. The basic versions of most sleep diary applications are free, but have premium subscription offers for advanced features that range from approximately $4 to $12 per month.

Strengths and Limitations

Sleep diaries have several advantages. They are convenient, unobtrusive, and inexpensive or free (e.g., Short et al., 2017). When completed daily, they reduce recall bias (Reda, 2015) that may be problematic with other subjective reports of sleep quality and quantity (Freedman et al., 1999). Finally, the promising psychometric properties of sleep diaries adds to their clinical utility.

The major limitation of the sleep diary is the lack of standardization. The lack of standardization hampers the ability to integrate and compare findings for sleep-related outcomes across studies (Carney et al., 2012). Reporter accuracy is another limitation (Short et al., 2013; Short et al., 2017; Werner et al., 2008). Because it is standard practice for caregivers to be the primary sleep diary informant (Spruyt & Gozal, 2011b), and caregivers tend to overestimate children's total sleep times (Dayyat et al., 2011; Short et al., 2013; Werner et al., 2008) and are often unaware of night awakenings (Werner et al., 2008), validity is likely compromised.

Finally, daily completion of sleep diaries can be burdensome (Galland et al., 2014; Sadeh, 2008; Thurman et al., 2018). Likewise, non-compliance has the potential to introduce error if completion of the measure is delayed by several days (Thurman et al., 2018). Research has suggested that individual factors such as parental fatigue (Sadeh, 1994) and personality characteristics like behavioral avoidance (Thurman et al., 2018) are associated with poorer compliance on sleep diaries. Furthermore, studies have also found that individual compliance with sleep diary completion diminishes significantly over time, meaning the longer one must complete the diary, the less reliable the data (Sadeh, 1994; Short et al., 2013; Thurman, 2018). Given the popularity of sleep diaries in intervention research and clinical care, efforts should be made to address the issue of burden; some researchers have found calling daily for the data, despite putting the burden on the researcher, improves compliance and data reliability (Kaier et al., 2020).

Child Considerations

When setting up sleep diary assessment with children and adolescents, practitioners should consider 1) who is going to be the most reliable and accurate reporter and 2) how to support families in regular completion of the diaries. Regarding the first consideration, practitioners should be mindful of the child's age when designating the primary reporter. Adolescents tend to be better reporters on sleep diaries when compared to parents. For children school-aged and younger, parents should consult with their child when completing – particularly because parents tend to overestimate total sleep duration. In order to promote regular sleep diary completion, practitioners should engage families in problem solving at the outset in order to preempt any barriers to success. This preventative approach might look like identifying a time of day for families to complete the sleep diary and even encouraging families to set an alarm as a reminder. Note, ideally the selected time will be shortly after awakening in order to prevent recall bias. Additionally, practitioners might help families select a location for the diary that will cue the family to complete it; being visible and convenient (e.g., on a fridge door or on the bathroom mirror) can increase compliance. Practitioners can also encourage families to use reinforcers at home to help facilitate compliance (e.g., sticker chart with prizes) and the practitioner might also consider implementing a reward system within their offices if feasible, so that when children return the completed diary they receive an small prize. Finally, collecting the data over the phone or using some other electronic device, so that a prompt or reminder cues the family to record the day's data can be helpful for increasing daily compliance.

QUESTIONNAIRES

The growing recognition and acceleration of pediatric sleep research has led to an expansion in the development of survey instruments and questionnaires. These questionnaires cover a range of sleep-related topics including sleep-wake patterns, sleep behaviors (e.g., snoring, insomnia), sleep problems, sleep habits, circadian cycles, dreams and nightmares, and daytime sleepiness (Spruyt & Gozal, 2011b). Questionnaire formats vary, but most are characterized by self-report or caregiver proxy forms and questions are asked using a variety of rating-type scales assessing frequency and severity of sleep-related concerns (Spruyt & Gozal, 2011b).

Spruyt and Gozal (2011b) published a comprehensive review of current pediatric sleep instruments. Their search yielded 183 pediatric sleep instruments, 57 of which were found to have been psychometrically evaluated to some degree. The majority of these 57 tools (k = 43, where k is number instruments) were published after the year 2000. In contrast, only two tools were published prior to 1980, two were published in the 1980s, and 10 were published in the 1990s. Over half of the tools were from the United States of America (k = 29), followed by Italy (k = 6), the United Kingdom (k = 5), Canada (k = 3), Australia (k = 3), and China (k = 3). The greatest proportion of these tools (k = 30) were implemented exclusively in community-school settings, with sample sizes ranging from 20 to 6,631 participants. Based on their lower age bound, seven tools were applicable as early as infancy, seven tools were for toddlers, 11 tools were for preschoolers, 22 tools were for school-aged children, nine tools were for early adolescence, of which two were applicable to middle adolescents. More than half of reviewed tools (k = 36) were parental report instruments. Across reviewed measures, the number of items ranged from 6 to 140, with 12 of these instruments reporting the estimated time to completion. The measures created for infancy were found to primarily concentrate on the sleep environment and soothing. Those instruments pertaining to preschool and school-aged children focused on sleep-wake patterns as well as sleep behaviors such as snoring and bedtime resistance. Adolescent measures were found to contain more questions regarding daytime sleepiness, circadian cycles, and emotional well-being. The timeframe evaluated ranged from 1 week up to a year; specifically, 15 tools covered 1 month, 9 tools assessed 6 months, and approximately 17 papers failed to report the period during which sleep was evaluated. Approximately 38 of reviewed questionnaires used solely closed-ended questions, with frequency ratings or a Likert-scale being the most commonly used response format. Noteworthy, the authors found that open-ended questions from interviews were seldomly psychometrically evaluated.

In their review, Spruyt and Gozal (2011b) concluded that only two of the 57 measures were suitably developed and psychometrically appropriate. Their judgement was based on an 11-step guide for the development and evaluation of subjective pediatric sleep assessment tools (Spruyt & Gozal, 2011a). For the current chapter, we will review the two instruments that Spruyt and Gozal determined were sufficiently developed: 1) The Sleep

Disorders Inventory for Students: Children and Adolescent Form (SDIS) and 2) the Sleep Disturbance Scale for Children (SDSC).

The SDIS arose from a Ph.D. dissertation in collaboration with an expert sleep panel and seven pediatric sleep centers in four regions of the United States (Luginbuehl et al., 2008). The SDIS was implemented with both a clinical and community sample consisting of 821 total children from diversified family demographics that reflected the 2000 census. The SDIS was refined through several stages. The SDIS was developed as a parent-report screening tool and has two forms, one for children aged 2 through 10 years and the other for adolescents aged 11 through 18 years (Luginbuehl, 2004). The instrument is comprised of five subscales representing five sleep disorders: obstructive sleep apnea, narcolepsy, periodic limb movement disorder, restless legs syndrome, and delayed sleep phase syndrome. There are 43 total items, which are rated on 7-point scale questioning frequency of behavior over the past 6 to 12 months. The measure takes approximately 10 minutes to complete. Spanish versions of the instruments are available; notably, two Spanish-speaking professionals translated the measures to ensure accuracy in terminology for Spanish-speaking families to complete (Luginbuehl et al., 2008). Overall, the measure demonstrated adequate internal consistency, and test-retest reliability as well as appropriate concurrent validity when scores were compared to sleep specialists' diagnoses of sleep disorders.

The SDSC was developed for children aged 3 to 18 years (Romeo et al., 2013) and is completed by the parent or caregiver. Its subscales assess disorders of initiating and maintaining sleep, disorders of arousal, sleep-wake transition disorders, disorders of excessive sleepiness and hypersomnolence (Bruni et al., 1996). These subscales are consistent with the categories of Association of Sleep Disorders Centers and the Association for the Psychophysiological Study of Sleep (1979) diagnostic classification of sleep and arousal disorders. The instrument includes 26-items, which are rated on a 5-point rating scale covering the last 6 months; it takes approximately 10 minutes to complete. There are multiple translations of the SDSC (Ferreira et al., 2009; Saffari et al., 2014) and the measure has been psychometrically validated for Brazilian Portuguese (Ferreira et al., 2009),

Italian (Bruni et al., 1996), and Belgian (Spruyt et al., 2004) populations. For example, the modified version of SDSC for Brazilian Portuguese families included written and visual communication of the measurement items and standardized explicit repetition of the subject for all items to accommodate reading abilities (Ferreira et al., 2009). Evidence suggests the measure is reliable and valid (Bruni et al., 1996). The SDSC was distributed to the primary caregivers of 1304 children (1157 controls) aged 6 to 15 years. The internal consistency was acceptable for the control group (Cronbach's alpha = .71) and for the sleep disordered group (Cronbach's alpha = .79); the test-retest reliability was adequate for the total score (r = .71). Additionally, factor analyses (variance explained 44.21%) yielded six factors which represented the most common areas of sleep disorders in childhood and adolescence. The re-evaluation of the sample, using the factor scores, supported the validity and the discriminating capacity of the scales between controls and the clinical groups.

Clinical Indications

Questionnaires are often the first phase of assessment for pediatric sleep concerns and inform decision making for further assessment and evaluation. In a clinical context, questionnaires are used as routine screening tools for a range of sleep parameters in pediatric populations (Honaker & Meltzer, 2016). Positive screens may initiate follow-up for specific diagnoses of common sleep disturbances in children, including difficulties initiating or maintaining sleep, excessive daytime sleepiness, snoring or other breathing problems, and abnormal movements before or during sleep (Wise & Glaze, 2019). Using questionnaires to screen children not only clarifies the presence or absence of sleep disturbances but can also inform frequency and severity of sleep concerns. Notably, only psychometrically sound instruments can accurately detect sleep problems, improve clinical decision making, and reduce errors in judgement (Spruyt & Gozal, 2011a).

Costs

The cost of questionnaires varies. Some questionnaires, such as the SCSC, are free to access and use by professionals and researchers. Other questionnaires, such as the SDIS, may be purchased by professionals or parents. Professionals can purchase the SDIS in large quantities, with costs ranging from $0.60 to $1.50 per screener, depending on the amount ordered (Child Uplift, Inc, 2018). In contrast, parents may purchase a single SDIS and complete the questionnaire for $14.95. Furthermore, cost for accessing and using questionnaires may vary based on author permission rights and publisher agreements.

Strengths and Limitations

There are both advantages and limitations to using pediatric sleep questionnaires. Current instruments are vast and readily available to practitioners and researchers. Furthermore, questionnaires provide efficient administration, convenience, and are a cost-effective solution to evaluate sleep parameters (Spruyt & Gozal, 2011b).

Regarding limitations, it is concerning that with the proliferation of available instruments, many lack sound psychometric properties, particularly with respect to validity evidence, and have not undergone thorough and careful construction (Lewandowski et al., 2011; Luginbuehl & Kohler, 2009; Spruyt & Gozal, 2011). Psychometrically insufficient instruments result in poor quality data, misleading conclusions, and inappropriate recommendations, and are therefore, highly problematic in both research and clinical care.

Additionally, there is currently no subjective instrument that can be applied exclusively to diagnose sleep disorders in pediatric populations (Bruni et al., 1996; Romeo et al., 2013). Diagnostic instruments allow for efficient and valid assignment of diagnosis and are necessary for both epidemiological research and clinical care. Also concerning, few if any measures utilize an interview response format; thereby increasing the likelihood that rater bias interferes with the accuracy of reporting. That is, parents might respond inaccurately by minimizing, exaggerating, or inconsistently reporting on their children's sleep behaviors, and closed-ended questions cannot query for cultural differences in normative sleep-related behaviors.

Although the SDIS and SCSC have cultural adaptations, Spruyt and Gozal (2011b) underscored that many questionnaires do not. The paucity of culturally sensitive pediatric sleep questionnaires is problematic because these tools are extensively used in both research and clinical care (Spruyt & Gozal, 2011b). Without culturally sensitive instruments, it is possible that sleep problems are being overlooked in certain groups of children. Given these limitations, future instrumentation should prioritize validation, rigorous development, creation of child and caregiver versions, diagnostic utility, protections from response bias, and cultural adaptations in order to advance the field of subjective pediatric sleep measurement.

Child Considerations

It is important to identify from the outset who is completing the questionnaire, either the caregiver on behalf of the child or the child independently. Most measures rely on caregivers as the primary informant. It is advantageous to have caregivers report on certain sleep parameters, particularly when dealing with preschool and school-aged children who are limited in their ability to reliably report on psychological symptoms (Edelbrock et al., 1985; Herjanic et al., 1975). However, evidence suggests that school-aged children over 8 years can be accurate reporters of sleep habits and sleep disturbances (Owens et al., 2000) and that adolescents are better informants of their sleep-wake patterns than their parents (Dayyat et al., 2011). As such, it is recommended to consider the child's developmental age to determine their ability to reliably complete questionnaires.

SUMMARY AND RECOMMENDATIONS FOR THE FUTURE

Pediatric sleep tools, both objective and subjective methods, are varied in both scope and number. The most commonly applied methods are polysomnography, actigraphy, sleep diaries, and questionnaires. Table 1 identifies these methods while summarizing their strengths and limitations. Polysomnography is considered the gold standard in pediatric sleep assessment (Marcus, 2001) because it is valid in detecting several specific sleep disorders, particularly those related to disordered breathing (Beck & Marcus, 2009) and it has standardized scoring criteria (Iber & Iber, 2007). However, PSG is expensive (American Sleep Association, 2019), taxing for both families and personnel (Beck & Marcus, 2009), challenging to administer to young children (Beck & Marcus, 2009; Zaremba et al., 2005), and can result in invalid reading on the first night of assessment (Agnew et al., 1966). Actigraphy is a cost-effective, convenient, and unobtrusive alternative objective sleep measure and is useful for identifying sleep-wake patterns (Martin & Hakim, 2011). However, actigraphy lacks standardization (Meltzer & Westin, 2011; Meltzer et al., 2012), is prone to over-estimating wakefulness (Galland et al., 2014), and may be burdensome for families due to the standard requirement for concurrent sleep diary completion.

Provided the inherent limitations of these objective tools with respect to cost, convenience, and scope, subjective measures like sleep diaries and questionnaires can be advantageous to use when evaluating sleep. Both sleep diaries and questionnaires are unobtrusive, often free or inexpensive (e.g., Short et al., 2017), and some have promising psychometric properties (Werner et al., 2008). Sleep diaries have the added benefit of minimizing the risk of recall bias because of their prospective response format (Reda, 2015). Questionnaires are easily accessible to clinicians and researchers and can inform decision making for further assessment of sleep concerns (Spruyt & Gozal, 2011b). While there are unique advantages for sleep diaries and questionnaires, by and large, both have limited psychometric properties and lack complete diagnostic coverage for all forms of youth sleep pathology. Sleep diaries lack a consistent, standardized format (Carney et al., 2012) and daily compliance can be burdensome (Galland et al., 2014; Sadeh, 2008; Thurman et al., 2018). Questionnaires have not yet undergone rigorous test construction (Spruyt & Gozal, 2011b) and rely on caregivers as the primary informant (Spruyt & Gozal, 2011b).

Having summarized the strengths and limitations of both objective and subjective sleep assessment tools, it is evident that research is needed to develop measures that are psychometrically valid, diagnostically comprehensive, and culturally sensitive. Given that many sleep disorders present with overlapping symptomology and that comorbidities are common, a single measurement tool that can comprehensively and simultaneously assess multiple types of pediatric sleep pathologies would have clinical utility. Structured clinical interviewing is a method that is commonly used to concurrently assess multiple types of psychopathology. This measurement approach is considered the gold standard for evaluating mental disorders in clinical research (APA Work Group on Psychiatric Evaluation, 2016; Rogers, 2001). To date, a structured clinical interview for pediatric sleep disorders does not exist. However, the authors of this chapter are currently developing a structured clinical interview for pediatric sleep disorders, which we anticipate will be available in 2022. This instrument will evaluate six of the most common sleep disorder diagnoses affecting children and adolescents - insomnia, hypersomnolence disorder, delayed sleep-wake phase disorder, non-REM sleep arousal disorder, nightmare disorder, and restless legs syndrome – and will screen for narcolepsy, and obstructive sleep apnea hypopnea. It is our hope that development of this tool will not only help facilitate accurate diagnosis and guide evidence-based treatment selection but will also help standardize and advance treatment research and epidemiology in the field of pediatric sleep medicine. We plan to design this instrument with the limitations of current subjective sleep instruments in mind, prioritizing cultural sensitivity and adhering to the rigorous construction guidelines published by Spruyt and Gozal (2011a).

Table 1. Summary of strengths and limitations for pediatric sleep assessment tools

Measure	Strengths	Limitations
Polysomnography	• Gold standard objective too[11] • Valid for specific diagnoses[2] • Standardized scoring criteria[3]	• Expensive[4] • Time- and labor-intensive[2] • Challenging to administer to young children[2] • Accuracy threatened by the first night effect[5]
Actigraphy	• Affordable[6] • Sensitive in detecting sleep periods[7]	• Poor specificity (i.e., over-identifies wakefulness)[7] • Requires complimentary sleep diary recordings[8] • Inefficient[9] • No standardized scoring or definitional critieria[7]
Sleep Diary	• Unobtrusive[10] • Free[10] • Promising psychometrics[11] • Reduces risk of recall bias[12]	• Heterogenous and non-standardized[13] • Burdensome[8] • Subject to inaccurate ratings based on informant[10, 11]
Questionnaire	• Time-effective[14] • Easily accessible[14] • Cover a range of sleep metrics[14] • Free or inexpensive[14]	• Paucity of culturally sensitive tools[14] • Inadequate psychometric properties[14] • Poorly constructed[15] • Lack diagnostic utility[14]

Note. [1]Marcus, 2001, [2]Beck & Marcus, 2009, [3]Iber & Iber, 2007, [4]American Sleep Association, 2019, [5]Agnew et al., 1966, [6]Martin & Hakim, 2011, [7]Meltzer et al., 2012, [8]Galland et al., 2014, [9]Acebo et al., 1999, [10]Short et al., 2017, [11]Werener et al., 2008, [12]Reda, 2015, [13]Carney et al., 2012, [14]Spruyt & Gozal, 2011b, [15]Spruyt & Gozal, 2011a.

REFERENCES

Acebo, C., & LeBourgeois, M. K. (2006). Actigraphy. *Respiratory Care Clinics of North America*, *12*(1), 23–30, viii. https://doi.org/10.1016/j.rcc.2005.11.010.

Acebo, C., Sadeh, A., Seifer, R., Tzischinsky, O., Wolfson, A. R., Hafer, A, & Carskadon, M. A. (1999). Estimating sleep patterns with activity monitoring in children and adolescents: How many nights are necessary for reliable measures? *Sleep, 22*(1), 95–103. http://dx.doi.org/10.1093/sleep/22.1.95.

Achenbach, T. M. (1991). *Manual for the Child Behavior Checklist, 4–18 and 1991 Profile.* University of Vermont, Department of Psychiatry.

Agnew Jr, H. W., Webb, W. B., & Williams, R. L. (1966). The first night effect: An EEG study of sleep. *Psychophysiology, 2*(3), 263-266. http://dx.doi.org/10.1111/j.1469-8986.1966.tb02650.x.

American Academy of Sleep Medicine. (2007). *The AASM manual for the scoring of sleep and associated events: Rule, terminology and technical specifications.* Association for the Psychophysiological Study of Sleep.

American Sleep Association (2019). *Home sleep test and sleep apnea sleep study testing.* Retrieved from https://www.sleepassociation.org/sleep-disorders/sleep-apnea/home-sleep-test-sleep-apnea-testing/.

American Sleep Disorders Association. (1997). Practice parameters for the indications for polysomnography and related procedures. *Sleep, 20*(6), 406-22.

Ancoli-Israel, S., Cole, R., Alessi, C., Chambers, M., Moorcroft, W., & Pollak, C. P. (2003). The role of actigraphy in the study of sleep and circadian rhythms. *Sleep, 26*(3), 342-392. doi: 10.1093/sleep/26.3.342

APA Work Group on Psychiatric Evaluation (2016). *Practice guidelines for psychiatric evaluation of adults.* American Psychiatric Association.

Aurora, R. N., Lamm, C. I., Zak, R. S., Kristo, D. A., Bista, S. R., Rowley, J. A., & Casey, K. R. (2012). Practice parameters for the non-respiratory indications for polysomnography and multiple sleep latency testing for children. *Sleep, 35*(11), 1467-1473. https://doi.org/10.5665/sleep.2190

Association of Sleep Disorders Centers. (1979). *Diagnostic classification of sleep and arousal disorders.* Raven.

Beck, S. E., & Marcus, C. L. (2009). Pediatric polysomnography. *Sleep Medicine Clinics, 4*(3), 393–406. http://dx.doi.org/10.1016/j.jsmc.2009.04.007.

Brockmann, P. E., Perez, J. L., & Moya, A. (2013). Feasibility of unattended home polysomnography in children with sleep-disordered breathing. *International Journal of Pediatric Otorhinolaryngology, 77*(12), 1960-1964. doi: 10.1016/j.ijporl.2013.09.011.

Bruni, O., Ottaviano, S., Guidetti, V., Romoli, M., Innocenzi, M., Cortesi, F., & Giannotti, F. (1996). The Sleep Disturbance Scale for Children (SDSC) Construction and validation of an instrument to evaluate sleep disturbances in childhood and adolescence. *Journal of Sleep Research, 5*(4), 251-261. http://dx.doi.org/10.1111/j.1365-2869.1996.00251.x.

Buysse, D. J., Ancoli-Israel, S., Edinger, J. D., Lichstein, K. L., & Morin, C. M. (2006). Recommendations for a standard research assessment of insomnia. *Sleep, 29*(9), 1155-1173. http://dx.doi.org/10.1093/sleep/29.9.1155.

Carney, C. E., Buysse, D. J., Ancoli-Israel, S., Edinger, J. D., Krystal, A. D., Lichstein, K. L., & Morin, C. M. (2012). The consensus sleep diary: Standardizing prospective sleep self-monitoring. *Sleep, 35*(2), 287-302. http://dx.doi.org/10.5665/sleep.1642.

Child Uplift, Inc (2018). *Sleep disorders inventory for students* (SDIS). http://www.sleepdisorderhelp.com/index.cfm?ID=7.

Conners, C. K. (1970). Symptom patterns in hyperkinetic, neurotic, and normal children. *Child Development, 41*(3), 667-682. http://dx.doi.org/10.2307/1127215.

Dayyat, E. A., Spruyt, K., Molfese, D. L., & Gozal, D. (2011). Sleep estimates in children: Parental versus actigraphic assessments. *Nature & Science of Sleep, 3*, 115–123. http://dx.doi.org/10.2147/NSS.S25676.

Edelbrock, C., Costello, A. J., Dulcan, M. K., Kalas, R., & Conover, N. C. (1985). Age differences in the reliability of the psychiatric interview of the child. *Child Development, 56*(1), 265-275. http://dx.doi.org/10.2307/1130193.

Ferreira, V. R., Carvalho, L. B., Ruotolo, F., de Morais, J. F., Prado, L. B., & Prado, G. F. (2009). Sleep Disturbance Scale for Children: Translation, cultural adaptation, and validation. *Sleep Medicine, 10*(4), 457-463. http://dx.doi.org/10.1016/j.sleep.2008.03.018.

Freedman, N. S., Kotzer, N., & Schwab, R. J. (1999). Patient perception of sleep quality and etiology of sleep disruption in the intensive care unit. *American Journal of Respiratory & Critical Care Medicine, 159*(4), 1155-1162. http://dx.doi.org/10.1164/ajrccm.159.4.9806141.

Galland, B., Meredith-Jones, K., Terrill, P., & Taylor, R. (2014). Challenges and emerging technologies within the field of pediatric actigraphy. *Frontiers in Psychiatry, 5,* 1-5. http://dx.doi.org/10.3389/fpsyt.2014.00099.

Galland, B. C., Short, M. A., Terrill, P., Rigney, G., Haszard, J., Coussens, S., Foster-Owens, M., and Biggs, S. N. (2018). Establishing normal values for pediatric nighttime sleep measured by actigraphy: A systematic review and meta-analysis. *Sleep, 41*(4), 1-16. https://doi.org/10.1093/sleep/zsy017.

Herjanic, B., Herjanic, M., Brown, F., & Wheatt, T. (1975). Are children reliable reporters? *Journal of Abnormal Child Psychology, 3*(1), 41-48. http://dx.doi.org/10.1007/BF00916029.

Honaker, S. M., & Meltzer, L. J. (2016). Sleep in pediatric primary care: A review of the literature. *Sleep Medicine Reviews, 25,* 31-39.

Iber, C., & Iber, C. (2007*). The AASM manual for the scoring of sleep and associated events: rules, terminology and technical specifications* (Vol. 1). American Academy of Sleep Medicine.

Irwin, M. R., Cole, J. C., & Nicassio, P. M. (2006). Comparative meta-analysis of behavioral interventions for insomnia and their efficacy in middle-aged adults and in older adults 55+ years of age. *Health Psychology, 25*(1), 3-14. http://dx.doi.org/10.1037/0278-6133.25.1.3.

Kaier, E., Rischard, M., Barlaan, D., & Cromer, L.D. (2020). *Reaching a rural community: Feasibility of delivering a child posttraumatic nightmare treatment via televideoconferencing* [Manuscript in preparation]. Department of Psychology, The University of Tulsa.

Katz, E. S., Greene, M. G., Carson, K. A., Galster, P., Loughlin, G. M., Carroll, J., & Marcus, C. L. (2002). Night-to-night variability of polysomnography in children with suspected obstructive sleep apnea. *The Journal of Pediatrics, 140*(5), 589-594. http://dx.doi.org/10.1067/mpd.2002.123290.

Lewandowski, A. S., Toliver-Sokol, M., & Palermo, T. M. (2011). Evidence-based review of subjective pediatric sleep measures. *Journal of Pediatric Psychology, 36*(7), 780-793. http://dx.doi.org/10.1093/jpepsy/jsq119.

Luginbuehl, M. L. (2004). The initial development and validation study of the Sleep Disorders Inventory for Students. *Dissertation Abstracts International Section A: Humanities & Social Sciences, 64*(12-A), 4376.

Luginbuehl, M., Bradley-Klug, K. L., Ferron, J., Anderson, W. M., & Benbadis, S. R. (2008). Pediatric sleep disorders: Validation of the sleep disorders inventory for students. *School Psychology Review, 37*(3), 409.

Luginbuehl, M., & Kohler, W. C. (2009). Screening and evaluation of sleep disorders in children and adolescents. *Child & Adolescent Psychiatric Clinics of North America, 18*(4), 825-838. http://dx.doi.org/10.1016/j.chc.2009.04.012.

Marcus, C. L. (2001). Sleep-disordered breathing in children. *American Journal of Respiratory & Critical Care Medicine, 164*(1), 16-30. http://dx.doi.org/10.1164/ajrccm.164.1.2008171.

Martin, J. L., & Hakim, A. D. (2011). Wrist actigraphy. *Chest, 139*(6), 1514-1527. http://dx.doi.org/10.1378/chest.10-1872.

Meltzer, L. J., Montgomery-Downs, H. E., Insana, S. P., & Walsh, C. M. (2012). Use of actigraphy for assessment in pediatric sleep research. *Sleep Medicine Reviews, 16*(5), 463-475. http://dx.doi.org/10.1016/j.smrv.2011.10.002.

Meltzer, L. J., & Westin, A. M. (2011). A comparison of actigraphy scoring rules used in pediatric research. *Sleep Medicine, 12*(8), 793-796. http://dx.doi.org/10.1016/j.sleep.2011.03.011.

Morin, C. M., Culbert, J. P., & Schwartz, S. M. (1994). Non-pharmacological interventions for insomnia: A meta-analysis of treatment efficacy. *American Journal of Psychiatry, 151*(8), 1172-1180. http://dx.doi.org/10.1176/ajp.151.8.1172.

Newell, J., Mairesse, O., Verbanck, P., & Neu, D. (2012). Is a one-night stay in the lab really enough to conclude? First-night effect and night-to-night variability in polysomnographic recordings among different clinical population samples. *Psychiatry Research, 200*(2-3), 795-801. http://dx.doi.org/10.1016/j.psychres.2012.07.045.

Owens, J. A., Spirito, A., McGuinn, M., & Nobile, C. (2000). Sleep habits and sleep disturbance in elementary school-aged children. *Journal of Developmental & Behavioral Pediatrics, 21*(1), 27-36. http://dx.doi.org/10.1097/00004703-200002000-00005.

Reda, F. (2015). Diagnostic tools and testing in the sleepless and restless patient. In R. K. Malhotra (Ed.), *Sleepy or Sleepless* (pp. 107-111). Springer International Publishing.

Rogers, A. E., Caruso, C. C., & Aldrich, M. S. (1993). Reliability of sleep diaries for assessment of sleep/wake patterns. *Nursing Research, 42*(6), 368-371. http://dx.doi.org/10.1097/00006199-199311000-00010.

Rogers, R. (2001). *Handbook of diagnostic and structured interviewing.* Guilford Press.

Romeo, D. M., Bruni, O., Brogna, C., Ferri, R., Galluccio, C., De Clemente, V., Di Jorio, M., Quintiliani, M., Ricci, D., & Mercuri, E. (2013). Application of the sleep disturbance scale for children (SDSC) in preschool age. *European Journal of Pediatric Neurology, 17*(4), 374-382. http://dx.doi.org/10.1016/j.ejpn.2012.12.009.

Sadeh, A. (1994). Assessment of intervention for infant night waking: parental reports and activity-based home monitoring. *Journal of Consulting & Clinical Psychology, 62*(1), 63-68. http://dx.doi.org/10.1037/0022-006X.62.1.63.

Sadeh, A. (2008). Commentary: Comparing actigraphy and parental report as measures of children's sleep. *Journal of Pediatric Psychology, 33*(4), 406-407. http://dx.doi.org/10.1093/jpepsy/jsn018.

Sadeh, A. (2015). III. Sleep assessment methods. *Monographs of the Society for Research in Child Development, 80*(1), 33-48. http://dx.doi.org/10.1111/mono.12143.

Sadeh, A., & Acebo, C. (2002). The role of actigraphy in sleep medicine. *Sleep Medicine Reviews, 6*(2), 113-124. http://dx.doi.org/10.1053/smrv.2001.0182.

Saffari, M., Gholamrezaei, A., Saneian, H., Attari, A., & Bruni, O. (2014). Linguistic validation of the Sleep Disturbance Scale for Children

(SDSC) in Iranian children with Persian language. *Sleep Medicine*, *15*(8), 998-1001. http://dx.doi.org/10.1016/j.sleep.2014.03.021.

Scholle, S., Scholle, H. C., Kemper, A., Glaser, S., Rieger, B., Kemper, G., & Zwacka, G. (2003). First night effect in children and adolescents undergoing polysomnography for sleep-disordered breathing. *Clinical Neurophysiology*, *114*(11), 2138-2145. http://dx.doi.org/10.1016/S1388-2457(03)00209-8.

Short, M. A., Arora, T., Gradisar, M., Taheri, S., & Carskadon, M. A. (2017). How many sleep diary entries are needed to reliably estimate adolescent sleep? *Sleep*, *40*(3), zsx006. http://dx.doi.org/10.1093/sleep/zsx006.

Short, M. A., Gradisar, M., Lack, L. C., Wright, H. R., & Chatburn, A. (2013). Estimating adolescent sleep patterns: Parent reports versus adolescent self-report surveys, sleep diaries, and actigraphy. *Nature & Science of Sleep*, *5*, 23-26. http://dx.doi.org/10.2147/NSS.S38369.

Smith, M. T., Perlis, M. L., Park, A., Smith, M. S., Pennington, J., Giles, D. E., & Buysse, D. J. (2002). Comparative meta-analysis of pharmacotherapy and behavior therapy for persistent insomnia. *American Journal of Psychiatry*, *159*(1), 5-11. http://dx.doi.org/10.1176/appi.ajp.159.1.5.

Spruyt, K., Cluydts, R., & Verleye, G. B. (2004). Pediatric sleep disorders: Exploratory modulation of their relationships. *Sleep*, *27*(3), 495-501. https://doi.org/10.1093/sleep/27.3.495.

Spruyt, K., & Gozal, D. (2011a). Development of pediatric sleep questionnaires as diagnostic or epidemiological tools: A brief review of dos and don'ts. *Sleep Medicine Reviews*, *15*(1), 7-17. http://dx.doi.org/10.1016/j.smrv.2010.06.003.

Spruyt, K., & Gozal, D. (2011b). Pediatric sleep questionnaires as diagnostic or epidemiological tools: A review of currently available instruments. *Sleep Medicine Reviews*, *15*(1), 19-32. http://dx.doi.org/10.1016/j.smrv.2010.07.005.

Stewart, S. A., Penz, E., Fenton, M., & Skomro, R. (2017). Investigating cost implications of incorporating level III at-home testing into a polysomnography based sleep medicine program using administrative data. *Canadian Respiratory Journal*, 1-7. https://doi.org/10.1155/2017/8939461.

Stone, K. L., & Ancoli-Israel, S. (2011). *Actigraphy – An Overview* (M. H. Kyger, T. Roth, & W. C. Dement Eds). Elsevier Inc.

Thurman, S. M., Wasylyshyn, N., Roy, H., Lieberman, G., Garcia, J. O., Asturias, A., Okafor, G. N., Elliott, J. C., Giesbrecht, B., Grafton, S. T., Mednick, S. C., & Vettel, J. M. (2018). Individual differences in compliance and agreement for sleep logs and wrist actigraphy: A longitudinal study of naturalistic sleep in healthy adults. *PloS One, 13*(1), e0191883. http://dx.doi.org/10.1371/journal.pone.0191883.

Werner, H., Molinari, L., Guyer, C., & Jenni, O. G. (2008). Agreement rates between actigraphy, diary, and questionnaire for children's sleep patterns. *Archives of Pediatric & Adolescent Medicine, 162*(4), 350–358. http://dx.doi.org/10.1001/archpedi.162.4.350.

Wise, M. S., & Glaze, D. G. (2019). Assessment of sleep disorders in children. In A. G. Hoppin (Ed.), *UpToDate*. Retrieved June 23, 2019, from https://www.uptodate.com/contents/assessment-of-sleep-disorders-in-children.

Zaremba, E. K., Barkey, M. E., Mesa, C., Sanniti, K., & Rosen, C. L. (2005). Making polysomnography more "child friendly:" A family-centered care approach. *Journal of Clinical Sleep Medicine, 1*(02), 189-198. http://dx.doi.org/10.5664/jcsm.26315.

In: Children and Sleep
Editor: Olivie Gadbois

ISBN: 978-1-53618-074-9
© 2020 Nova Science Publishers, Inc.

Chapter 2

SLEEP DISORDERS IN PEDIATRIC POPULATIONS: CLINICAL FEATURES, ETIOLOGIES, COMORBIDITIES, AND RULE-OUTS

Mollie E. Rischard[*], Devin R. Barlaan and Lisa D. Cromer, PhD
Department of Psychology,
The University of Tulsa, Tulsa, OK, US

ABSTRACT

Pediatric sleep disorders are varied and complex, which can impede accurate detection. The present chapter reviews the most common sleep disorders affecting children and adolescents. Specifically, this chapter unpacks the complexities of these pathologies by discussing the child-specific features, etiology, common comorbidities, and differential diagnostic considerations pertinent for each disorder.

---

[*] Corresponding Author's Email: mer597@utulsa.edu.

SLEEP DISORDERS IN PEDIATRIC POPULATIONS

According to epidemiological research, 25% to 40% of children and adolescents meet criteria for a sleep-related diagnosis (Owens, 2005). However, in primary care settings, only 4% of children are identified as having a sleep disorder (Meltzer et al., 2010; Rosen et al., 2001). There is a problem of under-identification of sleep disorders (Meltzer et al., 2010) largely due to the complexities of co-morbidities and rule-out considerations. Furthermore, there is a great deal of symptom overlap between sleep disorders and other mental health conditions, which can mask sleep disorders (Owens, 2001). Behavioral manifestations of sleep disturbances include inattention, hyperactivity, emotional dysregulation, and academic failures; these symptoms may be misdiagnosed as other types of pathology, such as attention deficit hyperactivity disorder (ADHD; Yoon et al., 2012), learning disorders (Dewald et al., 2010), or some other mental disorder (Chervin et al., 2003).

The purpose of this chapter is to review the complexities of pediatric sleep pathologies by describing the most common DSM-5 sleep disorders affecting pediatric populations: insomnia, hypersomnolence disorder, narcolepsy, obstructive sleep apnea hypopnea, circadian rhythm sleep-wake disorders – delayed sleep phase type, non-rapid eye movement sleep arousal disorder, nightmare disorder, and restless legs syndrome. Each disorder reviewed in this chapter will include a description of diagnostic criteria, followed by developmental considerations and child-specific features of the disorder including unique clinical presentations at various ages, etiology, common comorbidities, and differential diagnostic considerations (see Tables 1.1 and 1.2 respectively for a summary). The chapter will conclude by discussing recommendations for the detection of sleep pathologies in pediatric healthcare settings.

INSOMNIA DISORDER

Insomnia disorder is characterized in the DSM-5 as one having difficulties initiating and/or maintaining sleep, and usually includes extended periods of nocturnal wakefulness and/or insufficient sleep quantity (APA, 2013). In order to meet diagnostic criteria, insomnia symptoms must occur at least 3 days a week for at least 3 months and represent a predominant complaint that is not fully explained by another medical condition (APA, 2013). Co-occurring medical (e.g., pain), psychiatric (e.g., depression), and/or other sleep disorders (e.g., sleep-disordered breathing) can be coded as unique specifiers rather than exclusions for diagnosis (APA, 2013). When insomnia is secondary to another condition, an insomnia diagnosis is recommended only when the insomnia is sufficiently severe to warrant independent clinical attention (APA, 2013). There are various categorizations of this disorder (APA, 2013). Sleep onset insomnia, or initial insomnia, involves difficulty falling asleep at bedtime. Sleep maintenance insomnia, or middle insomnia, involves frequent and/or prolonged night awakenings. Late insomnia entails early-morning awakenings with an inability to return to sleep. These combinations of sleep difficulties occur despite adequate opportunity and time for sleep and result in some form of daytime impairment (APA, 2013). Research with adults has found that the onset of insomnia symptoms can occur at any point in life, but the first episode typically occurs during young adulthood (Bastien et al., 2004).

Prevalence

Insomnia has been reported to affect anywhere from 4% to 41% of children and adolescents (Owens, 2019). Studies with school-aged children (ages 5-12 years) have discovered prevalence rates as high as 30% based on parental reports of children's difficulties falling asleep and staying asleep (Calhoun et al., 2014). Studies on insomnia disorder in adolescents have found prevalence rates ranging from 8% (Dohnt et al., 2012) to 19% (Hysing et al., 2013) with up to 36% experiencing insomnia-related symptoms several times a month (Laberge et al., 2001). There is an increased prevalence of insomnia in girls compared to boys, with differences typically emerging after the onset of puberty (Calhoun et al., 2014; Ohayon et al., 2000).

Etiology

Pediatric insomnia is typically the result of a combination of intrinsic and extrinsic factors (Owens, 2019). Intrinsic factors are those that are innate or unique to the child that predispose them to sleep problems (Owens, 2019). These factors include having a first-degree family member affected by insomnia (APA, 2013), anxious or difficult temperament, medical issues (e.g., chronic pain, headaches), neurodevelopmental disorders (e.g., autism, intellectual disabilities, and ADHD), and psychiatric comorbidities (e.g., anxiety and depression). Insomnia with pubertal onset is associated with circadian preferences, affecting teens who are "night owls" or "morning larks." Extrinsic factors that impact insomnia onset are environmental stimuli that precipitate and/or perpetuate the onset of sleep struggles (Owens, 2019). These may be parenting practices such as poor limit-setting (e.g., allowing a teen to stay up until 2 a.m. playing video games on a school night) or developmentally inappropriate expectations about bedtimes (e.g., expecting a teen to observe the same bedtime as a much younger sibling). Poor sleep environments can also contribute to insomnia onset (Owens, 2019). Examples of poor sleep environments include a bed crowded with pets or toys, a room that is too hot or which has poor light or noise control, sharing sleeping quarters with snorers, or a household or neighborhood that is generally loud and disruptive.

Pediatric Clinical Features

Difficulties initiating and maintaining sleep are the most commonly reported complaints for youth populations, but clinical presentations of insomnia vary by age and developmental periods (Vriend & Corkum, 2011). For toddlers and young children, behavioral insomnia, which is characterized by a refusal to comply with bedtime, is one of the most common concerns, affecting approximately 20% to 30% of this age group (Honaker & Meltzer, 2014). Manifestations of behavioral insomnia usually resemble a child procrastinating going to bed. A child might demonstrate outright noncompliance to parental requests to get ready for bed either directly with a verbal refusal, or indirectly, by playing, using electronics, or reading instead of getting ready for bed. Some children's bedtime resistance occurs by way of dependence on the parent for the child to fall asleep; for example, a 5-year-old who needs a back rub to fall asleep, or a 10-year- old who needs a parent to lay down with them until the child is asleep (Vriend & Corkum, 2011). Some clinicians have coined the term "curtain calls," to characterize frequent requests for parental attention following lights out, which can delay the child's sleep onset by 30 minutes or more (Mindell & Owens, 2015, p. 77). Refusals that are powerfully reinforced, for example, with backrubs or other forms of comfort, quickly can manifest into chronic problems. Refusals and requests for attention after the child's bedtime should not be confused with a bedtime routine that may include healthy forms of comfort and attachment. For example, a healthy, adaptive bedtime routine may well include cuddles and stories as the child is getting ready for bed. The refusal is identified when it is not part of the pre-bedtime routine, but rather occurs as a form of delay or avoidance. It is important to distinguish between a bedtime routine and behavioral insomnia or bedtime stalling due to nighttime fears (e.g., fear of the dark). Behavioral insomnia often is associated with evening stress for the family and with frequent night awakenings (Vriend & Corkum, 2011).

For older children and adolescents, psychophysiological, or conditioned, insomnia is more common than behavioral insomnia (Owens, 2019). This presentation is characterized by anxiety about falling or staying asleep. Specifically, individuals experience heightened physiological and emotional arousal related to sleep and the sleep environment, which is believed to be the result of faulty conditioning, such that the bed is associated with wakefulness rather than sleepiness (Harvey, 2002). This conditioning is typically a corollary of behavioral insomnia. The child who was afraid of the dark, and who had no opportunity to learn an alternative association of the dark, experience the bed or sleep environment as a fear trigger. If for example, they never fell asleep with the light off, or without a parent comforting them, when they have a normal night awakening in the sleep cycle, the child could be hyper-aroused and unable to self-soothe or go back to sleep. Conditioned insomnia is often accompanied by maladaptive cognitions about the consequences of sleep problems that exacerbate one's ability to sleep (Harvey, 2002). For example, when awakening at 2 a.m., catastrophic thinking about not being able to get back to sleep and worrying about being tired for a test the next day, would contribute to one's insomnia cycle.

Rule-Out Considerations

There are several conditions that should be ruled out prior to diagnosing pediatric insomnia. Delayed sleep wake phase disorder (DSWPD), which is incongruence between the bedtime required by external circumstances and the child's natural sleep onset time, could manifest as insomnia symptoms (Chang et al., 2009). Insomnia can be distinguished from DSWPD when there are persistent sleep onset difficulties event after a schedule resumes in which the child or adolescent can select their bedtime. For example, if a child does not experience the sleep difficulties during spring break when they set their own schedule, insomnia would be ruled out. Although nighttime fears and separation anxiety could develop into delayed sleep onset insomnia, if the child can fall asleep with comfort, for example, when a transitional object or parent is present, insomnia would not be diagnosed (Muris et al., 2001). Transient or adjustment-related insomnia would not qualify for an insomnia diagnosis unless the symptoms persisted for at least one month (Owens & Mindell, 2011). Transient or adjustment-related insomnia is insomnia that occurs in response to a stressful event, change in sleeping environment (e.g., moving), disruption of sleep schedule due to jet lag, or due to an illness. Children with restless legs syndrome (RLS) also often present with sleep onset difficulties; however, these symptom presentations are uniquely characterized by an irresistible urge to move the extremities so RLS would be the appropriate diagnosis rather than insomnia, if other insomnia features were not present (Picchietti et al., 2007). Medication side effects can also masquerade as insomnia, so examining when insomnia symptoms emerged is important. If, for example, sleep problems began after a child started steroids or stimulant medications, an insomnia diagnosis would not be rendered without first ruling out that it was not a medication side effect. Anxiety-related disorders and/or ritualistic behaviors associated with obsessive compulsive disorders may also result in delayed sleep onset that is typical of insomnia. In these cases, insomnia should only be diagnosed if the sleep disturbance caused by the anxiety and/or ritualistic behaviors was severe enough to warrant clinical attention (Owens & Mindell, 2011).

HYPERSOMNOLENCE DISORDER

Hypersomnolence is a broad diagnostic term in which the principal complaint is excessive daytime sleepiness (APA, 2013). In order to meet criteria for hypersomnolence disorder, the excessive sleepiness should not be attributed to disturbed nocturnal sleep or misaligned circadian rhythms (APA, 2013). There are three primary symptoms of hypersomnolence disorder (APA, 2013). The first symptom is excessive quantity of sleep characterized by extended nocturnal sleep (>9 hours) and/or involuntary daytime sleep. The second is decreased quality of wakefulness as shown by difficulty awakening or inability to remain awake in situations that demand wakefulness (e.g., in the classroom). The third symptom of hypersomnolence is sleep inertia, which is characterized as a "sleep drunkenness," whereby an individual may demonstrate extreme confusion, irritability, or even aggression upon forced awakening (APA, 2013, p. 369). The symptom patterns for hypersomnolence disorder must occur at least 3 days a week for at least a 3 month period and should be accompanied by significant distress or daytime impairment in order to be diagnosed (APA,

2013). Individuals with this disorder often have short sleep latencies, falling asleep soon after going to bed, and can easily remain asleep throughout the night.

Prevalence

According to the DSM-5 (APA, 2013), approximately 5%-10% of adults who consult sleep disorder clinics with complaints of daytime sleepiness are diagnosed with hypersomnolence disorder. While excessive daytime sleepiness is estimated to occur in approximately 10% to 20% of school-aged and adolescent children (Calhoun et al., 2011), prevalence rates for hypersomnolence diagnoses are not available for pediatric populations and cases are reportedly rare (APA, 2013; Mindell & Owens, 2015). Although full manifestation of the disorder generally emerges in late adolescence, with symptoms typically beginning between ages 15 and 25 years (Ali et al., 2009), the disorder often goes undiagnosed for 10-15 years after symptom onset (APA, 2013). Research has not examined gender and/or sex differences for the disorder in pediatric populations, however, female adolescents tend to exhibit higher rates of daytime sleepiness in comparison to male adolescents (Lee et al., 1999).

Etiology

Although hypersomnolence disorder is poorly understood (Billiard, 2007), its etiology is believed to involve a combination of both environmental and genetic/physiological factors (Billiard & Sonka, 2016). A high proportion of hypersomnolence cases seem to run in families (Ali et al., 2009; Anderson et al., 2007; Billiard & Dauvilliers, 2001). However, researchers caution that more rigorous studies with clinical interviews and sleep studies in relatives are warranted in order to support a hereditary relationship (Billiard & Sonka, 2016). Physiological stress and substance use can temporarily increase hypersomnolence (APA, 2013). Additionally, damage to the central nervous system can trigger onset of hypersomnolence (Billiard & Sonka, 2016). Such damage can occur from illnesses like viral infections and metabolic disorders, and from neurological disorders, such as head trauma resulting from concussions (Billiard & Sonka, 2016).

Pediatric Clinical Features

In pediatric populations with hypersomnolence complaints, excessive daytime sleepiness is often the chief concern (Thomas & Burgers, 2018). The overwhelming urge to fall asleep is more pronounced during periods of inactivity, such as while watching a movie or sitting through a lecture. Sleep attacks may also occur; a sleep attack could be a brief microsleep lasting several seconds (Frucht et al., 1999), or one could last up to 90 minutes (Mindell & Owens, 2015). These episodes are often accompanied by sleep inertia complaints. In other words, if an involuntary nap occurs, it is later followed by difficulty falling asleep at night. Microsleeps can be difficult to diagnose if a parent does not witness them, because individuals with hypersomnolence are often unaware of experiencing microsleeps. Microsleeps are recognized by others who may notice that the child stares off in a daze or is unresponsive; microsleeps can go undetected when they occur while a child is engaging in an automatic or repetitive behavior.

Paradoxically, young children with hypersomnolence may have increased motor activity and behavioral disinhibition when they are excessively drowsy (Stores et al., 2006). These behaviors may be interpreted by healthcare professionals as inattentiveness or hyperactivity related to ADHD (Stores et al., 2006). Onset of sleepiness is often abrupt and profound, although it may improve over time, and may present as extended need for nocturnal sleep and/or regular and prolonged daytime napping (Fallone et al., 2002). Teachers are often the first professionals to note and report these problems because of the excessive daytime sleepiness observed in the classroom (Fallone et al., 2005).

Rule-Out Considerations

Several differential conditions should be ruled out before diagnosing hypersomnolence disorder. Insufficient sleep is the primary cause of excessive drowsiness in children and adolescents (Thomas & Burgers, 2018). Behaviorally induced insufficient sleep syndrome is characterized by an inadequate amount of nocturnal sleep (<7 hours per night) due to personal choices and can produce excessive sleepiness that resembles hypersomnolence disorder (Khan & Trotti, 2015). Therefore, amount of time the child sleeps is crucial for distinguishing between these two disorders. Individuals with breathing-related sleep disorders may also present with hypersomnolence complaints but can be differentiated from those with hypersomnolence disorder based on reports of loud snoring or pauses in breathing during sleep (APA, 2013). Parasomnias, a collection of disorders involving regular night awakenings and circadian-rhythm sleep-wake disorders, which are characterized by abnormal sleep-wake schedules, may also contribute to excessive sleepiness and should be considered as primary diagnoses (Dye et al., 2015). Narcolepsy and hypersomnolence share the core symptom of excessive daytime sleepiness but are distinct based on several key features. Individuals with hypersomnolence typically have longer periods of uninterrupted nocturnal sleep, greater difficulty waking, more persistent daytime drowsiness, and longer and less-restorative daytime naps with little or no dreaming (Ahmad et al., 2019). As will be reviewed below, a defining feature of narcolepsy that distinguishes it from other sleep disorders, is that many patients experience cataplexy. Certain mental disorders, like depression, may be associated with excessive daytime sleepiness (Dauvilliers et al., 2013). In these cases, if hypersomnolence symptoms represent the primary complaint, then hypersomnolence disorder may be diagnosed in addition to the depression or other associated disorder (APA, 2013). Certain substances can cause excessive sleepiness. Thus, prior to diagnosing hypersomnolence disorder, examiners should review medications and substance use as potential causes (APA, 2013).

NARCOLEPSY

Narcolepsy is another disorder in which the central feature is daytime sleepiness. Patients with narcolepsy experience recurrent episodes of an irrepressible need to sleep, lapses into sleep, or napping, and there may be multiple episodes in each day (APA, 2013). A unique feature of narcolepsy is cataplexy, which is a sudden loss of muscle tone when experiencing emotional duress or excitement (Lowenfeld, 1902). Emotional triggers of cataplexy can be positive (e.g., laughter) or negative, (e.g., stress or anger). Anticipatory anxiety or embarrassment can also trigger cataplexy (Anic-Labat et al., 1999). Situational triggers for cataplexy could include being startled, tickled, strong emotional memories, being the center of attention, or hearing something funny (Anic-Labat, et al., 1999). Although cataplexy involves partial loss of voluntary muscle control, it does not involve loss of consciousness. Interestingly however, individuals may be unaware of an episode of cataplexy when it is as subtle as tingling, twitching, or dropping things (Anic-Labat et al., 1999). In children, cataplexy often presents as spontaneous grimaces or jaw-opening episodes without an emotional trigger (Nevsimalova, 2014).

Other features of narcolepsy include possible sleep paralysis, characterized by the inability to move or speak for a few seconds or minutes after sleep onset or offset, and hypnagogic hallucinations, which are vivid, frightening dream-like experiences that occur during sleep onset and offset (Akintomide & Rickards, 2011). Affected individuals have confirmed deficiencies in hypocretin, also referred to as orexin, which is the hormone that promotes wakefulness (APA, 2013). Lab tests to confirm the hypocretin deficiency help with definitive diagnosis. Polysomnography is also generally required when diagnosing narcolepsy. Narcolepsy is a lifelong sleep disorder (Akintomide & Rickards, 2011).

Prevalence

The prevalence rate of pediatric narcolepsy is unknown because it develops gradually and is under-identified (Nevsimalova, 2014). In adults, the prevalence is less than 1% of the population (Ohayon et al., 2002; Silber et al., 2002). Like hypersomnolence disorder, symptoms typically emerge in late adolescence (Nevsimalova, 2014).

Etiology

Narcolepsy develops as a result of both environmental and genetic factors. Eight to 10% of patients with narcolepsy have a family member with the disorder (Mignot, 1998). Several winter-borne infections, such as streptococcal infections and influenza are associated with narcolepsy onset (Aran et al., 2009; Natarajan et al., 2013). Autoimmune diseases, such as multiple sclerosis, Cron's disease, and ulcerative colitis, are considered likely precipitators of the autoimmune process responsible for producing the orexin deficits characteristic of narcolepsy (APA, 2013; Akintomide & Rickards, 2011).

Pediatric Clinical Features

Children with narcolepsy often experience significant psychological distress associated with the functional impairment related to the excessive sleepiness (Inocente et al., 2014; Stores et al., 2006). Affected youth often present with a decreased quality of life, impaired academic performance, and significant concerns of safety (e.g., car accidents) due to excessive sleepiness and risk of sleep attacks (Inocente et al., 2014). Narcolepsy is often comorbid with migraines, obesity, early-onset puberty, and with other sleep disorders such as obstructive sleep apnea and periodic limb movement disorder in children (Nevsimalova, 2014). Psychiatric comorbidities include depression and anxiety in youth populations (Inocente et al., 2014).

Rule-Out Considerations

There are several differential diagnoses to consider when assessing for narcolepsy. Narcolepsy and hypersomnolence are both characterized by excessive daytime sleepiness; however, unlike hypersomnolence, individuals with narcolepsy also have confirmed insufficiencies of hypocretin and/or cataplexy. Temporary sleep deprivation and insufficient nocturnal sleep could be implicated in extreme drowsiness and should first be ruled out. Sleep apnea syndromes (Alexander & Schroeder, 2013) and depression (Dauvilliers et al., 2013) are associated with excessive daytime sleepiness, however, if cataplexy is present, narcolepsy should be considered as a comorbid diagnosis. Because sleepiness can cause increased motor activity in children, narcolepsy might appear as ADHD symptomology (Nevsimalova, 2014). Cataplexy can also be misidentified as a seizure disorder, conversion disorder, chorea, or other movement disorder (Guilleminault & Pelayo, 2000). Finally, schizophrenia can be misidentified when hypnagogic hallucinations are present; if cataplexy is endorsed, the clinician should assume these symptoms are explained by narcolepsy before considering a co-occurring diagnosis of schizophrenia (Talih, 2011).

OBSTRUCTIVE SLEEP APNEA HYPOPNEA

Obstructive sleep apnea hypopnea (OSAH) is the most common of all respiratory sleep disorders (APA, 2103) and when undetected and untreated, can be dangerous (Carroll & Loughlin, 1995). OSAH is characterized by repeated episodes of prolonged partial airway obstruction and/or intermittent complete airway obstruction during sleep, and is accompanied by respiratory effort (APA, 2013). Apnea refers to the total absence of airflow, and hypopnea refers to a reduction in airflow (APA, 2013). This obstruction in airflow can lead to reduced oxygen intake during sleep and/or awakenings during sleep episodes (Carroll & Loughlin, 1992). For children with OSAH, breathing obstruction is often caused by enlarged tonsils and/or adenoids, which results in raspy breathing or light snoring in young children and loud snoring in older children (Carroll & Loughlin, 1995). Snoring and daytime sleepiness are the cardinal symptoms of OSAH (APA, 2013). Polysomnography or a sleep study is required for diagnosis (Beck & Marcus, 2009).

Prevalence

There is considerable research on rates of pediatric OSAH. For children under 8 years of age, the prevalence is approximately 2.5% (Marcus, 2001) and OSAH affects about 6% of adolescents (Johnson & Roth, 2006). The development and course of the disorder mirrors a J-shaped distribution (APA, 2013), with a peak in onset between ages 3-8 years when the upper airway may be compromised with a relatively large mass of tonsillar tissue (APA, 2013). There is a decline in OSAH prevalence later in childhood when the airway develops. Prevalence rates sharply spike (thus the "J" shape) in post-pubertal adolescents due to increases in obesity rates at this stage of development (Chang & Chae, 2010).

Etiology

There is an amalgam of demographic, physiological, and genetic risk factors for OSAH. OSAH has a genetic basis (Chang & Chae, 2010). Parents of children with OSAH self-report symptoms of OSA at rates of 4% to 11% (Lumeng & Chervin, 2008). OSAH is more common in boys than girls (Sanchez-Armengol et al., 2008) and in African American children than in Caucasian children (Rosen et al., 2001). Upper airway obstruction due to a range of physiological factors, like asthma (Narayanan et al., 2019) or displacement of major facial structures (Cakirer et al., 2001), can predispose a child to OSAH. Medical conditions, such as Down's Syndrome (Chamseddin et al., 2019), obesity (Narayanan et al., 2019), and premature birth (Rosen et al., 2001) and environmental factors, such as exposure to secondhand smoke (Groner et al., 2019) and living in poverty (Spilsbury et al., 2006), also increase the risk for OSAH.

Pediatric Clinical Features

For pediatric populations, OSAH presentations vary by age, but typically consist of both nocturnal and daytime symptoms. Nighttime signs of the disorder include loud, continuous snoring, apneic pauses, which can appear as gasping, choking, or snoring during the night, and paradoxical movement of the chest and abdomen, meaning that during inspiration, the chest contracts, and during expiration, it expands (Alexander & Schroeder, 2013). Restless sleep, such as thrashing and increased body movement, as well as sweating, and mouth breathing while asleep, are also signs of OSAH (Chang & Chae, 2010). Daytime physical symptoms manifest in multiple ways, including mouth breathing and complaints of dry mouth, chronic nasal congestion, hyponasal speech, morning headaches, frequent infections such as sinusitis, difficulty swallowing, and poor appetite (Alexander & Schroeder, 2013). Children with the disorder often present with excessive daytime sleepiness, mood instability, internalizing concerns like somatic complaints, as well as externalizing behaviors such as aggression and impulsivity (Alexander & Schroeder, 2013). Additionally, there is a substantial overlap between the clinical impairment caused by OSAH and the diagnostic criteria for ADHD, including inattention, poor concentration, hyperactivity, and poor peer relations (Sedky et al., 2014). Academic and cognitive problems, such a poor executive functioning, are also often present in children with OSAH (Luo et al., 2019). Finally, OSAH is associated with a number of other disorders and conditions in pediatric populations, including enuresis (Weintraub et al., 2013), growth failure (Bonuck et al., 2006), increase in partial arousal parasomnias (Owens et al., 1997), increased seizure frequency for children with epilepsy (Rodriguez, 2007), and other comorbid sleep problems (Alexander & Schroeder, 2013).

Rule-Out Considerations

When confronted with features of OSAH, there are several conditions to rule out before diagnosing the disorder. One of these differentials includes primary snoring, which is otherwise known as snoring in the absence of key OSAH symptoms determined by polysomnography (Alexander & Schroder, 2013). Additionally, narcolepsy, circadian rhythm sleep disorders, and insomnia, which can also cause daytime sleepiness, also should be ruled out (Alexander & Schroder, 2013). Nocturnal panic attacks may include symptoms of gasping and choking that mimic OSAH presentations but can be distinguished based on the unpredictability and lower frequency of the episodes (Craske & Tsao, 2005). As mentioned, ADHD symptomology often resembles the clinical impairment from OSAH; however, research has indicated that ADHD symptomology decreases significantly when children with OSAH undergo adenotonsillectomy (Sedky et al., 2014). Finally, sleep related movements mimicking OSAH-related gasping and arousals may occur with nocturnal seizures and periodic limb movement disorder (APA, 2013). Thus, these disorders should be ruled out prior to diagnosing OSAH.

CIRCADIAN RHYTHM SLEEP-WAKE DISORDER - DELAYED SLEEP PHASE TYPE

The most common type of circadian rhythm sleep-wake disorder in pediatric populations is delayed sleep wake phase disorder (DSWPD; Nesbitt, 2018). Circadian rhythm disorders are characterized by a persistent and recurrent pattern of sleep disruption that is due to a misalignment between a person's natural circadian rhythm and the sleep-wake schedule required by their physical environment (APA, 2013). This disruption leads to excessive sleepiness during the day and causes clinically significant distress or impairment (APA, 2013). DSWPD is primarily characterized as a delay in the major sleep period by at least two hours resulting in insufficient sleep due to the wake time necessitated by environmental demands being two hours too early (Nesbitt, 2018). This is common in shift workers and in children and adolescents who are required to get up earlier than their bodies' natural rhythms call for, due to early school start times, early practice times for athletes, and the like (Nesbitt, 2018). The individual's body is unable to adjust to the schedule needed and cannot fall asleep early enough to get sufficient sleep, but if they were able to sleep later, their bodies allow it. For example, a teenager may be unable to fall asleep at 9 p.m., and even if they try, they may be unable to fall asleep until 11 p.m., resulting in chronic sleep deprivation if they have to wake at 6 a.m. each school day.

Prevalence

Prevalence of DSWPD is less than 0.5% in adults. Seven to 16% of adolescents struggle with DSWPD (APA, 2013; Lovato et al., 2013). Onset is typically during adolescence when circadian preferences shift to later times (Bartlett et al., 2013). Although high rates of excessive daytime sleepiness are documented in student-athletes due to schedule demands (Kaier et al., 2016), rates of the disorder have not yet been documented in this population.

Etiology

Biological, environmental, and psychosocial factors contribute to the etiology and maintenance of DSWPD (Gradisar & Crowley, 2013b). Forty percent of individuals with DSWPD have a positive family history of the disorder (Carter et al., 2014). One of the most prominent predisposing biological factors for the diagnosis is a longer than average circadian period, such as delayed bedtimes and delayed weekend wake times (Saxvig et al., 2013). Another potentially important and overlooked biological contributor to DSWPD is a misalignment in the two-process model of sleep (Saxvig et al., 2013). The two-process model promotes sleep via 1) the accumulation of homeostatic pressure to feel tired during wakefulness and 2) the activation of the circadian process to experience sleep during the evening (Hagenauer et al., 2009). Thus, individuals with DSWPD are more likely have a slower accumulation of homeostatic pressure and delayed internal circadian process leading to a greater evening alertness (Hagenauer et al., 2009; Saxvig et al., 2013). Light sensitivity might also play a role (Watson et al., 2018). Individuals with DSWPD may be hypersensitive to evening light, which can serve as a delay signal to the circadian clock (Watson et al., 2018). Exposure to screens and other electronic devices can prevent the brain's natural release of melatonin and thus, may further contribute to the development and maintenance of the delayed sleep phase (Nesbitt, 2018). Environmental factors such as late evening activities and/or sports practice, as well as late-day caffeine consumption, may further delay sleep onset (Saxvig et al., 2012). Psychosocial factors include school-related pressures, such as early school start times, and increased social pressures to stay up late (Saxyig et al., 2012). Notably, engaging in social gatherings in the evening or staying up late completing academic responsibilities may be preferred, thus perpetuating delayed sleep and increasing difficulties going to sleep and waking up (Saxvig et al., 2012). Pre-sleep cognitive activity, such as intrusive and unhelpful racing thoughts during bedtime, is also implicated in the development of the disorder (Gradisar & Crowley, 2013a), especially the child worrying about how they will function if over-tired the next day (Hiller et al., 2014).

Pediatric Clinical Features

The most common presenting complaints of DSWPD in adolescents are delayed sleep onset and oversleeping/daytime sleepiness (Bartlett et al., 2013). Poor school attendance is also common. Additional symptoms include consistently late sleep onset, which is generally after midnight in adolescents, as well as minimal difficulty with sleep maintenance throughout the night (Bartlett et al., 2013). Adolescents with the disorder might also complain of significant difficulty waking up at the required time as well as significant difficulty falling asleep at an earlier time (Bartlett et al., 2013). Daytime sleepiness might express in the form of napping, inattention, and occasional bouts of dozing off (Heussler, 2005). Although less common in younger children, associated features of DSWPD for preschool and elementary aged children include bedtime resistance and delayed sleep onset, evening or night preference, oversleeping on the weekend, poor school performance, tardiness or absenteeism from school, and increased caffeine use (Scherrer et al., 2016; Wickersham, 2006).

Rule-Out Considerations

There are several differential conditions to consider when a child presents with DSWP complaints. Insomnia is also characterized by difficulties initiating sleep but is distinct from DSWPD in one clear way: individuals with insomnia experience difficulties initiating sleep no matter what time they go to bed (Chang et al., 2009). In contrast, individuals with DSWPD have no problems falling asleep if they go to bed at their body's programmed sleep-onset time. Additionally, restless legs syndrome, which is characterized by an irresistible urge to move the extremities and is accompanied by uncomfortable sensations in the legs that worsen during inactivity and relieve during movement, may also lead to delays in sleep onset (Picchietti et al., 2007); in these cases, restless legs syndrome would be the primary diagnosis. Poor sleep hygiene and evening screen time may also result in delayed sleep onset (Brown et al., 2002), however, a diagnosis of DSWPD is only warranted if delayed sleep onset persists even after correcting these poor sleep habits (APA, 2013). In cases of later circadian preference, or being a "night owl," DSWPD should be diagnosed when the symptoms are intractable, persistent, and are associated with impaired functioning (APA, 2013). Lifestyle issues, such as socializing and late-night gaming or television viewing, can also lead to insufficient sleep quantity and difficulty waking up in the morning, however, these cases would not qualify as DSWPD if difficulties achieving sleep onset are not present (Mindell & Owens, 2015; Saxvig et al., 2012). Children and adolescents with school avoidance or refusal, which can result from anxiety or learning disorders, can also present with delayed sleep onset and difficulty awakening. In these cases, DSWPD would only be diagnosed if the sleep schedule is intractable, and an appropriate sleep-wake schedule cannot be maintained on the weekends and holidays (APA, 2013; Saxvig et al., 2012). School avoidance commonly co-occurs with and exacerbates DSWPD. Other mental health disorders, like depression and anxiety, often involve difficulties achieving sleep onset, but the set sleep-wake pattern characteristic of DSWPD is typically not present in these other pathologies (Nesbitt, 2018). Notably however, DSWPD is strongly associated with depression and may be comorbid with depression (Glozier et al., 2014). Finally, substances and other medications can lead to insufficient sleep and daytime sleepiness and should be ruled out when considering a DSWPD diagnosis (Hasler et al., 2014).

PARASOMNIAS: NON-RAPID EYE MOVEMENT SLEEP AROUSAL DISORDER

Parasomnias are defined as unwanted physical events or experiences that occur during sleep onset, within sleep, or during sleep offset (Driver & Shapiro, 1993). Non-REM (NREM) sleep arousal disorder falls under this broader category of parasomnias. An individual with NREM sleep arousal disorder has incomplete arousals that begin within a few hours after sleep onset, and which occur during the slow wave sleep phase (APA, 2013). NREM sleep arousal episodes subsume sleep walking and sleep terrors. Sleepwalking involves rising from bed and walking about (APA, 2013). Although usually benign, sleep walking can be associated with safety concerns, such as walking outside or falling out of windows, and should be addressed if this is the case (Mason & Pack, 2007). Sleep terrors are characterized by an abrupt terror arousal, usually accompanied by a behavioral manifestation of fear, like a panicky sounding scream (APA, 2013). During the episode, the individual is often unconscious and therefore, typically appears inconsolable and unresponsive to the efforts of others to provide comfort (APA, 2013). The incomplete arousals characteristic of both sleepwalking and sleep terrors are typically brief, lasting 1 to 10 minutes, but may extend up to 1 hour (APA, 2013). The arousals are referred to as incomplete because they are characterized by amnesia for the episode (Bonkalo, 1974). During sleep walking and sleep terrors, it is difficult if not impossible to wake the individual, and if awakened, they typically are confused but not distressed (Bonkalo, 1974; Nguyen et al., 2008). When hearing about their night terror episode being recounted by someone else, it is common for those who have them to not only struggle recalling the episode, but to also to appear embarrassed. In contrast to a nightmare, in which suffers experience distress and/or dysphoria, sleep terrors are not associated with distress of those who experience them; however, family members, especially parents may be distressed from the screams or from having their own sleep disturbed. The frequency of both sleepwalking and sleep terrors range from a one-time event to a nightly occurrence, with some individuals experiencing multiple episodes in one night (Mindell & Owens, 2015).

Prevalence

NREM sleep arousal disorder is more frequent in childhood than in adolescence or adulthood. However, prevalence rates differ by the type of arousal episode with sleepwalking being more common than sleep terrors. Prevalence estimates for isolated instances of sleepwalking range from 15% to 40% for pediatric populations (Mason & Pack, 2007). Approximately 17% of youth sleepwalk regularly, with 3% to 4% of these youth reporting frequent episodes (Mason & Pack, 2007). Onset of sleepwalking is usually between 4 and 6 years, and peak frequency is between 8 and 12 years (Klackenberg, 1982). Regular episodes typically extend for a 5-year span before remitting (Klackenberg, 1982). Sleep terrors are rarer. Approximately 1% to 6.5% of children experience sleep terrors episodes, primarily during preschool and elementary school years (Mason & Pack,

2007). The age of onset is typically between ages 4 and 12 years (Mason, & Pack, 2007). Episodes are typically most frequent with onset and are generally more regular with a younger age of onset (Mason & Pack, 2007).

Etiology

Disorders of arousal are believed to be caused by several factors including genetic predispositions and irregularities in the sleep cycle progression (Mason & Pack, 2007). Regarding heritability, individuals who experience arousal episodes frequently have a positive family history of either sleep terrors or sleepwalking, with as high as a 10-fold increase in the prevalence of the disorder among first-degree biological relatives (APA, 2013). Pertaining to sleep cycle abnormalities, it is important to first distinguish between the two types of sleep: REM and NREM sleep. REM sleep is characterized by rapid eye movements, more dreaming and bodily movement, and faster pulse and breathing. Conversely, NREM sleep is considered by slow-wave and dreamless sleep, whereby breathing and heart rate are slow and regular, blood pressure is low, and the sleeper is relatively still. The comparative proportion of REM and NREM sleep changes throughout the night, such that NREM sleep typically predominates the first third of the night and REM sleep in the last third. For individuals with arousal disorders, the transition from NREM to REM sleep is abnormal and the individual is not fully awake or asleep (Mason & Pack, 2007). Children spend more time in NREM sleep than do adults, which explains the higher risk for the disorder in childhood (Mason & Pack, 2007). There are multiple other factors that may influence arousal episodes including medical and mental conditions, like migraines and Tourette syndrome (Mason & Pack, 2007). Additionally, there are several environmental factors that have been shown to trigger and/or exacerbate the arousal episodes. These include factors like sleep deprivation, irregular sleep schedule, shifts in sleep schedules, comorbid sleep disturbances like OSAH and restless legs syndrome, fever and illness, situational stress and anxiety, caffeine consumption, noise and light, and sleeping with a full bladder (Mason & Pack, 2007; Mindell & Owens, 2015).

Pediatric Clinical Features

NREM sleep arousal disorder is characterized by unique clinical features in pediatric populations (Irfan et al., 2017). Sleepwalking typically presents as a nocturnal episode that involves unusual or bizarre behavior, such as walking into a sibling's room or walking aimlessly thorough the house (Irfan et al., 2017). These episodes are often accompanied by confusion, agitation, and incoherent responses to questions (Irfan et al., 2017). Sleep terrors usually emerge abruptly and range from mild, whereby the child simply appears agitated and/or confused, to severe, in which the child is found crying and/or screaming (Irfan et al., 2017). Because these episodes often appear dramatic, parents may be concerned that the child has undergone a traumatic experience or that the episodes themselves are traumatic (Irfan et al., 2017). However, there is no evidence to suggest that these events are rooted in trauma or that they cause emotional distress (Stores, 2007). Nevertheless, parental anxiety about the arousal episodes is common in children presenting for treatment (Thiedke, 2001). NREM sleep problems may interfere with social functioning because of potential embarrassment, for example, a child may avoid sleepovers or summer camp (Stores, 2007).

Rule-Out Considerations

Clinicians should consider key differential diagnoses when presented with concerns of NREM sleep arousal disorder. Nocturnal seizures can often be challenging to distinguish from disorders of arousals (Zucconi & Ferini-Strambi, 2000). Major characteristics of seizure disorder include stereotypic or repetitive behaviors, multiple arousal events per night, occurrence of nighttime seizures during the sleep-wake transitions or after the first third of the night and associated daytime sleepiness (Zucconi & Ferini-Strambi, 2000).

Parents may label disorders of arousal as nightmares, so it is important to ask parents to characterize what they mean by nightmare (Mason & Pack, 2005). Disorders of arousal often occur during the first half of the night, often when parents are still awake, and the child has no or very limited recall of the event. On the other hand, nightmares often happen during the second half of the night and early morning when parents are asleep, and a child can typically recall explicit details from the dream and will remember the event the next day. A child will also be reluctant to return to sleep following a nightmare and might seek comfort from their caregiver. Finally, the features of nocturnal panic attacks often mimic those of arousal episodes (Stores, 2007). However, in cases of nocturnal panic attacks, the events can be recalled the next morning and there are often similar episodes that occur during the day (Craske & Tsao, 2005).

PARASOMNIAS: NIGHTMARE DISORDER

Nightmares are considered the second type of parasomnia and are thus classified under the parasomnia category of mental disorders when their frequency and severity reach the pathological threshold. This threshold necessitates repeated occurrences of dysphoric and well-remembered dreams that cause clinically significant distress or impairment (APA, 2013). These dreams typically cause awakening, and memory for dream content involve threats to survival, security, or physical integrity (APA, 2013). On awakening from the nightmare, an individual will rapidly become oriented and alert (APA, 2013). Nightmare frequency determines severity of the disorder; mild cases involve less than one episode per week, moderate cases involve one or more episodes per week, and severe cases involve nightly episodes (APA, 2013). Nightmares often occur in the second half of a sleep event, specifically and most commonly during REM sleep. Nightmares terminate upon awakening; however, the negative emotions may persist into wakefulness, making it difficult to return to sleep; they can also result in dysphoria during the day (APA, 2013). While nightmare content varies, it typically focuses on attempts to avoid or cope with imminent danger and may involve themes that evoke other unpleasant emotions, such as anger, disgust, embarrassment, or sadness (APA, 2013).

Prevalence

Experiencing occasional nightmares is quite common. Approximately 75% of children report having at least one nightmare in their lifetime (Gauchat et al., 2014). Rates of nightmare disorder within pediatric populations are unknown but are believed to be under-diagnosed. Cromer and colleagues (under review) found that of 822 pediatric psychiatry outpatients, only .01% had a diagnosis of nightmare disorder in their electronic medical record, yet 40% of patients they screened ($n = 622$) were positive for regular, recent, nightmare episodes. Further research has indicated that when chronic nightmares are defined as having more than one nightmare per month, prevalence ranges from 6% to 44% in adolescent populations (Gauchat et al., 2014). For very frequent nightmares, or instances in which children reported experiencing more than one nightmare per week, prevalence estimates differed across samples from 2% in children aged 5 to 18 years, to 2-4% in preschool children, to 19% in children aged 9 to 11 years (Gauchat et al., 2014). Peak nightmare prevalence is between ages 6 and 10 years for both boys and girls, after which time, girls generally report more nightmares (Gauchat et al., 2014).

Etiology

There are several factors that impact the development and exacerbation of nightmare disorder in children. Parental-endorsed nightmare prevalence has been linked with nightmares in children, which may be due to both environmental and hereditary factors (Reynolds & Alfano, 2015). Experiencing prior, isolated episodes of nightmares can put children at an increased risk for more chronic nightmare events (Schredl et al., 2009a). Stress and/or traumatic experiences, such as abuse, neglect, and exposure to violence, can trigger and intensify nightmare episodes (Secrist et al., 2019), as can anxiety (Schredl et al., 2009a; Secrist et al., 2019). Children who also reportedly experience insomnia or complaints of insufficient sleep are also more likely to report having nightmares (Li et al., 2011; Schredl et al., 2009a). Finally, medications, particularly those that have a direct impact on REM sleep, can also induce and/or exacerbate nightmare occurrence (Foral et al., 2011).

Pediatric Clinical Features

Nightmare content differs across ages and development (Stores, 2007). Young children's nightmare themes include separation anxiety or images of monsters and other scary creatures (Stores, 2007). For older children, nightmares might reflect frightening content for shows they have seen or books they have read, or actual disturbing daytime experiences (Stores, 2007). For children of all ages, nightmare onset may be contiguous to traumatic events or stressful experiences. In these cases, nightmares might replicate or resemble the events, or may be completely dissimilar (Gray & Cromer, 2018). Nightmares occurring after traumatic events are characterized as trauma-related, or posttraumatic nightmares, and are distinct from idiopathic nightmares, or nightmares of unknown origin (Langston et al., 2010). Trauma-related nightmares are associated with higher levels of distress and impairment than are idiopathic nightmares (Langston et al., 2010) and trauma-related nightmare content often reflects severe threats and contains more significant consequences than do idiopathic nightmares (Punamäki et al., 2005; Valli et al., 2006).

For pediatric populations, the functional impairment from chronic nightmares is seen in global and diffuse daytime fears and/or anxiety (Schredl et al., 2009b). Additionally, children might exhibit bedtime resistance or hyperactivity because they associate bedtime and sleep with nightmares (Reynolds & Alfano, 2015). Affected children might also be more likely to have daytime behavioral problems, such as emotional outbursts, mood disturbances, and poor academic performance because of the excessive daytime sleepiness resulting from their disrupted sleep episode (Li et al., 2011).

Rule-Out Conditions

There are several conditions to rule out when encountering presentations of nightmare disorders. Nightmares are an intrusion symptom of posttraumatic stress disorder (PTSD; APA, 2013) and acute stress disorder (ASD; APA 2013). Children may develop nightmares following a traumatic event and if nightmares were not previously present, a nightmare disorder would not be diagnosed secondary to the PTSD. Children with separation anxiety disorder (SAD) may experience repeated nightmares which, if not occurring before the development of SAD, would not be diagnosed in addition to the primary disorder of SAD (APA, 2013). Above and beyond nightmares being a part of the symptomatology of PTSD, ASD, and a common co-occurring feature of SAD, nightmares can also accompany several mental disorders, including insomnia, schizophrenia, personality disorders, as well as mood, anxiety, and adjustment-related disorders (Lemyre et al., 2019). In these cases, a concurrent nightmare diagnosis should only be considered when independent clinical attention is warranted, otherwise, no separate diagnosis is needed (APA, 2013). Regarding other diagnostic considerations, NREM sleep arousals, which include sleep terrors and sleepwalking, are often difficult for parents to distinguish from nightmares. Nightmares are distinct from arousal episodes based on several key features, including their occurrence in the second half of the sleep episode during REM sleep, vivid recollection of dream content, minimal confusion or disorientation upon awakening, and delayed return to sleep (Stores, 2007). Additionally, nocturnal seizures might appear similar to nightmare episodes; however, unlike nightmares, seizures often also include stereotypic or repetitive behaviors and other motor and sensory characteristics (Stores, 2007). Finally, REM behavior disorder is also characterized by experiences of violent and scary dreams; however, REM behavior disorder often involves complex motor activity during these dream episodes whereas nightmare episodes do not (APA, 2013).

RESTLESS LEGS SYNDROME

Restless legs syndrome (RLS) is a sensorimotor, neurological sleep disorder characterized by a strong urge to move one's legs and arms (Allen at al., 2003; APA, 2013). The urge is usually accompanied by uncomfortable sensations commonly described as creeping, crawling, tingling, burning, or itching (Allen at al., 2003; APA, 2013). These sensations are usually only partially relieved through continuous movement such as walking, rocking, stretching, and rubbing (Allen at al., 2003; APA, 2013). Most episodes begin or are exacerbated by inactivity (Allen at al., 2003; APA, 2013), such as lying in bed or riding in a car. There is a circadian component to the episodes, such that they typically peak in the evening hours (Allen at al., 2003). Thus, the conditions that worsen RLS are also the same conditions that promote sleep initiation: bedtime. Conversely, the behaviors that relieve RLS episodes are those that most impede sleep onset: movement. This symptom-relief cycle hinders children from achieving consistent, quality sleep. The diagnosis of RLS is based primarily on history and child self-report.

Prevalence

RLS is common in adults, with prevalence ranging from 5% to 10% (Allen et al., 2005; Bjorvatn et al., 2005; Högl et al., 2005). A history of childhood onset before the age of 10 years is present in approximately 8-13% of reported adult cases (Bassetti et al., 2001; Montplaisir et al., 1997; Walters et al., 1996). For pediatric populations, prevalence of the disorder ranges from 1% to 6% (Picchietti et al., 2007).

Etiology

There are several factors that increase the risk of RLS development and impact its maintenance. Overall, it is estimated that between 50% and 60% of individuals with RLS have a positive family history among first-degree relatives (Desai et al., 2004). Precipitating factors are typically time-limited, such as iron deficiency and pregnancy, with most individuals resuming normal sleep patterns after the trigger has resolved (APA, 2013; Durmer & Quraishi, 2011; Einollahi & Izadianmehr, 2014). Other chronic medical conditions, such as sickle cell disease, migraine headaches, diabetes, and pain syndromes are also associated with onset of RLS symptomology (Zucconi & Ferini-Strambi, 2004). Finally, insufficient sleep, certain medications, especially antihistamines and antidepressants, as well as excessive caffeine consumption may exacerbate underlying RLS (Durmer & Quraishi, 2011).

Pediatric Clinical Features

Children with RLS often report both an urge to move and discomfort in their legs. Descriptors children use include, "need to move," "got to kick," as well as being in "pain" or "hurting" (Picchietti et al., 2011). It is common for children with RLS to initially present with sleep disturbance difficulties, including bedtime resistance, delayed sleep onset, restless sleep, and night awakenings (Picchietti et al., 2013). However, above and beyond these sleep concerns, there are distinguishable features of RLS including a combination of motor, sensory, and daytime complaints in children. The sleep, motor, sensory, and daytime complaints are more likely to manifest as behavioral and educational concerns (Picchietti et al., 2013). Motor symptoms are expressed as restless leg movements during the daytime, as well as walking, pacing or running about during long periods of inactivity and during bedtime (Picchietti et al., 2013). Consequently, children with RLS may have difficulty staying in their seat at school and appear to have ADHD-like symptoms such as inattention, poor concentration, and distractibility (Durmer & Quraishi, 2011; Picchietti et al., 2013). Sensory symptoms are characterized as leg pain or discomfort during periods of inactivity and in the evening. Daytime complaints include excessive daytime sleepiness or fatigue, mood instability, and externalizing behaviors such as aggression and impulsivity (Durmer & Quraishi, 2011).

Rule-Out Conditions

There are number of pediatric conditions that appear to mimic RLS profiles and should be ruled out in RLS evaluations. Nocturnal leg discomfort or pain should be a primary differential consideration in presentations of RLS (Picchietti et al., 2013). Specific conditions might include nocturnal leg cramps (Durmer & Quraishi, 2011), exercise-related muscular pain, transient nerve compression such as the feeling of pins and needles following long periods of inactivity, growing pains, or nonspecific leg discomfort (Picchietti et al., 2013). It is important to differentiate that sore leg muscles often worsen with movement, whereas children with RLS will often experience relief with movement (Picchietti et al., 2013). These problems typically peak at bedtime and wake children from sleep (Piccietti et al., 2013). Sleep-related motor restlessness, which can be caused by problems like sleep apnea, parasomnias, or ADHD, should also be ruled out in cases of RLS-like complaints (Picchietti et al., 2013). Other associated features of RLS relate primarily to co-occurring mental health concerns, including hyperactivity, impulsivity, inattention, anxiety, and depression (Durmer & Quraishi, 2011; Picchietti et al., 2013). Furthermore, common RLS symptoms like prolonged sleep onset, nighttime awakening, and excessive daytime sleepiness could be attributed to a range of other issues such as behavior problems, OSAH, or DSWPD (Picchietti et al., 2013) so those problems should be ruled out.

CONCLUSION

In summary, sleep disorders are prevalent among pediatric populations (Owens, 2005). This chapter reviewed the eight most common DSM-5 sleep disorders affecting pediatric populations, including insomnia, hypersomnolence disorder, narcolepsy, obstructive sleep apnea hypopnea, circadian rhythm sleep-wake disorders – delayed sleep phase type, non-rapid eye movement sleep arousal disorder, nightmare disorder, and restless legs syndrome. Each pediatric sleep disorder discussed in this chapter identified prevalence, etiology, clinical features, and a summary of medical, sleep, and psychological rule-out considerations. Pediatric sleep pathologies present a complex constellation of symptoms and there is significant overlap between sleep disorders and other health conditions that often complicate assessment and identification of these disorders in healthcare settings (Meltzer et al., 2010; Owens, 2001). Provided these complexities, Tables 1.1 and 1.2 were created to summarize co-occurring conditions and rule-out considerations for pediatric sleep disorders.

A key theme that resonated throughout this review, is that patient's description of a problem (e.g., "night terror") may warrant further behavioral probes so that their labels do not mask the presence of an underlying disorder. When parents and children describe sleep problems, it will be important for clinicians to ask what that looks like, or what the patient means, when they say, for example, they have a night terror. Knowing when the child wakes, how they behave upon awakening, and what time of night the event takes place, can help with accurate diagnosis. Similarly, understanding the unique features and clinical presentations of sleep pathologies can help with accurate detection of sleep problems that could otherwise manifest as behavioral disorders (Ahmad et al., 2019).

Table 1.1. Summary of co-occurring conditions for pediatric sleep disorders

Sleep Disorder	Medical	Sleep	Psychological
Insomnia Disorder	• Medical issues (e.g., chronic pain; headaches) • Puberty	• Poor sleep hygiene	• Autism spectrum disorder • Intellectual disabilities • ADHD • Anxiety • Depression
Hypersomnolence Disorder			• Depression
Narcolepsy	• Migraines • Obesity • Precocious puberty	• Other sleep disorders (e.g., parasomnias)	• Bipolar disorder • Anxiety • Depression
Obstructive Sleep Apnea Hypopnea (OSAH)	• Growth failure • Seizures	• Other sleep problems (e.g, Nocturnal enuresis • NREM Sleep Arousals	
Circadian Rhythm Sleep-Wake Disorder: Delayed Sleep Wake Phase			• Anxiety • Depression • School avoidance
NREM Sleep Arousal Disorder	• Migraines • Tourette's syndrome	• OSAH	
Nightmare Disorder	• Medical conditions (e.g., chronic pain)	• Insomnia/ insufficient sleep	• Trauma exposure/PTSD • Anxiety • Depression • Adjustment disorder • Schizophrenia • Personality disorders
Restless Legs Syndrome	• Migraines • Sickle cell disease • Diabetes • Pain syndromes		• ADHD • Anxiety • Depression

Note. ADHD = Attention Deficit Hyperactivity Disorder. DSWPD = Delayed sleep wake phase disorder. OSAH = Obstructive sleep apnea hypopnea. RLS = Restless legs syndrome. PTSD = Posttraumatic stress disorder.

Table 1.2. Summary of rule-out considerations for pediatric sleep disorders

Sleep Disorder	Medical	Sleep	Psychological
Insomnia Disorder	• Medication effects	• Transient insomnia (e.g., jetlag) • Nighttime fears • DSWPD • RLS	• Separation anxiety • PTSD
Hypersomnolence Disorder	• Medication effects	• Insufficient sleep • Breathing-related sleep disorders • Parasomnias • Circadian-rhythm sleep-wake disorders	• ADHD • Depression • Trauma exposure
Narcolepsy	• Seizures • Movement disorders	• Insufficient sleep • Hypersomnolence disorder • Breathing-related sleep disorders	• ADHD • Depression • Schizophrenia
Obstructive Sleep Apnea Hypopnea (OSAH)	• Nocturnal seizures • Periodic limb movement disorder	• Primary snoring • Narcolepsy • Circadian Rhythm Sleep Disorders • Insomnia	• Nocturnal panic attacks • ADHD
Circadian Rhythm Sleep-Wake Disorder: Delayed Sleep Wake Phase	• Substance/medication use	• Poor sleep hygiene • Circadian preference • Insomnia • RLS	• School avoidance • Anxiety • Depression
NREM Sleep Arousal Disorder	• Nocturnal seizures	• Nightmares	• Nocturnal panic attacks
Nightmare Disorder	• Nocturnal seizures	• NREM sleep arousals • REM behavior disorder	• PTSD
Restless Leg Syndrome (RLS)	• Nocturnal leg discomfort/pain	• Sleep-related motor restlessness • OSAH • DSWPD	• Behavior issues

Note. ADHD = Attention Deficit Hyperactivity Disorder. DSWPD = Delayed sleep wake phase disorder. OSAH = Obstructive sleep apnea hypopnea. RLS = Restless legs syndrome. PTSD = Posttraumatic stress disorder.

REFERENCES

Ahmad, A. M. M., Sinniah, D., Habil, M. H., & How, S. L. (2019). A review on sleep-disorders in children and adolescents. *Asian Journal of Pediatric Research, 2*(3), 1-20. https://doi.org/10.9734/ajpr/2019/v2i330110.

Akintomide, G. S., & Rickards, H. (2011). Narcolepsy: A review. *Neuropsychiatric Disease & Treatment, 7*(1), 507-518. https://doi.org/10.2147/NDT.S23624.

Alexander, N. S., & Schroeder, J. W. (2013). Pediatric obstructive sleep apnea syndrome. *Pediatric Clinics, 60*(4), 827-840. https://doi.org/10.1016/j.pcl.2013.04.009.

Ali, M., Auger, R. R., Slocumb, N. L., & Morgenthaler, T. I. (2009). Idiopathic hypersomnia: Clinical features and response to treatment. *Journal of Clinical Sleep Medicine, 5*(06), 562-568. http://dx.doi.org/10.5664/jcsm.27658.

Allen, R. P., Picchietti, D., Hening, W. A., Trenkwalder, C., Walters, A. S., & Montplaisi, J. (2003). Restless legs syndrome: Diagnostic criteria, special considerations, and epidemiology: A report from the restless legs syndrome diagnosis and epidemiology workshop at the National Institutes of Health. *Sleep Medicine, 4*(2), 101-119. https://doi.org/10.1016/S1389-9457(03)00010-8.

Allen, R. P., Walters, A. S., Montplaisir, J., Hening, W., Myers, A., Bell, T. J., & Ferini-Strambi, L. (2005). Restless legs syndrome prevalence and impact: REST general population study. *Archives of Internal Medicine, 165*(11), 1286-1292. doi: 10.1001/archinte.165.11.1286.

American Psychiatric Association. (2013). *Diagnostic and statistical manual of mental disorders* (5th ed.). Author.

Anderson, K. N., Pilsworth, S., Sharples, L. D., Smith, I. E., & Shneerson, J. M. (2007). Idiopathic hypersomnia: A study of 77 cases. *Sleep, 30*(10), 1274-1281. http://dx.doi.org/10.1093/sleep/30.10.1274.

Anic-Labat, S., Guilleminault, C., Kraemer, H. C., Meehan, J., Arrigoni, J., & Mignot, E. (1999). Validation of a cataplexy questionnaire in 983 sleep-disorders patients. *Sleep,* 22(1), 77-87.

Aran, A., Lin, L., Nevsimalova, S., Plazzi, G., Hong, S. C., Weiner, K., Zeitzer, J., & Mignot, E. (2009). Elevated anti-streptococcal antibodies in patients with recent narcolepsy onset. *Sleep, 32*(8), 979-983. http://dx.doi.org/10.1093/sleep/32.8.979.

Bartlett, D. J., Biggs, S. N., & Armstrong, S. M. (2013). Circadian rhythm disorders among adolescents: assessment and treatment options. *Medical Journal of Australia, 199*(S8), S16-S20. https://doi.org/10.5694/mja13.10912.

Bassetti, C. L., Mauerhofer, D., Gugger, M., Mathis, J., & Hess, C. W. (2001). Restless legs syndrome: A clinical study of 55 patients. *European Neurology, 45*(2), 67-74. https://doi.org/10.1159/000052098.

Bastien, C. H., Vallieres, A., & Morin, C. M. (2004). Precipitating factors of insomnia. *Behavioral Sleep Medicine, 2*(1), 50-62. https://doi.org/10.1207/s15402010bsm0201_5.

Beck, S. E., & Marcus, C. L. (2009). Pediatric polysomnography. *Sleep Medicine Clinics, 4*(3), 393–406. http://dx.doi.org/10.1016/j.jsmc.2009.04.007.

Billiard, M. (2007). Diagnosis of narcolepsy and idiopathic hypersomnia. An update based on the International Classification of Sleep Disorders, 2nd Edition. *Sleep Medicine Reviews, 11*(5), 377-388. http://dx.doi.org/10.1016/j.smrv.2007.04.001.

Billiard, M., & Dauvilliers, Y. (2001). Idiopathic hypersomnia. *Sleep Medicine Reviews, 5*(5), 349-358. https://doi.org/10.1053/smrv.2001.0168.

Billiard, M., & Sonka, K. (2016). Idiopathic hypersomnia. *Sleep Medicine Reviews, 29*, 23-33. https://doi.org/10.1016/j.smrv.2015.08.007.

Bjorvatn, B., Leissner, L., Ulfberg, J., Gyring, J., Karlsborg, M., Regeur, L., Skeidsvoll, H., Nordhus, I. H., & Pallesen, S. (2005). Prevalence, severity and risk factors of restless legs syndrome in the general adult population in two Scandinavian countries. *Sleep Medicine, 6*(4), 307-312. https://doi.org/10.1016/j.sleep.2005.03.008.

Bonkalo, A. (1974). Impulsive acts and confusional states during incomplete arousal from sleep: Criminological and forensic implications.

Psychiatric Quarterly, *48*(3), 400-409. http://dx.doi.org/10.1007/BF01562162.

Bonuck, K., Parikh, S., & Bassila, M. (2006). Growth failure and sleep disordered breathing: A review of the literature. *International Journal of Pediatric Otorhinolaryngology, 70*(5), 769-778. https://doi.org/10.1016/j.ijporl.2005.11.012.

Brown, F. C., Buboltz Jr, W. C., & Soper, B. (2002). Relationship of sleep hygiene awareness, sleep hygiene practices, and sleep quality in university students. *Behavioral Medicine, 28*(1), 33-38. https://doi.org/10.1080/08964280209596396.

Cakirer, B., Hans, M. G., Graham, G., Aylor, J., Tishler, P. V., & Redline, S. (2001). The relationship between craniofacial morphology and obstructive sleep apnea in whites and in African-Americans. *American Journal of Respiratory & Critical Care Medicine, 163*(4), 947-950. https://doi.org/10.1164/ajrccm.163.4.2005136.

Calhoun, S. L., Fernandez-Mendoza, J., Vgontzas, A. N., Liao, D., & Bixler, E. O. (2014). Prevalence of insomnia symptoms in a general population sample of young children and preadolescents: Gender effects. *Sleep Medicine, 15*(1), 91-95. https://doi.org/10.1016/j.sleep.2013.08.787.

Calhoun, S. L., Vgontzas, A. N., Fernandez-Mendoza, J., Mayes, S. D., Tsaoussoglou, M., Basta, M., & Bixler, E. O. (2011). Prevalence and risk factors of excessive daytime sleepiness in a community sample of young children: The role of obesity, asthma, anxiety/depression, and sleep. *Sleep, 34*(4), 503-507. http://dx.doi.org/10.1093/sleep/34.4.503.

Carroll, J. L., & Loughlin, G. M. (1992). Diagnostic criteria for obstructive sleep apnea syndrome in children. *Pediatric Pulmonology, 14*(2), 71–74. http://dx.doi.org/10.1002/ppul.1950140202.

Carroll, J. L., & Loughlin, G. M. (1995). Obstructive sleep apnea syndrome in infants and children: Diagnosis and management. *Principles & practice of sleep medicine in the child*, 163-191.

Carter, K. A., Hathaway, N. E., & Lettieri, C. F. (2014). Common sleep disorders in children. *American Family Physician, 89*(5), 368-377.

Chamseddin, B. H., Johnson, R. F., & Mitchell, R. B. (2019). Obstructive sleep apnea in children with Down syndrome: Demographic, clinical, and polysomnographic features. *Otolaryngology–Head & Neck Surgery, 160*(1), 150-157. http://dx.doi.org/10.1177/0194599818797308.

Chang, S. J., & Chae, K. Y. (2010). Obstructive sleep apnea syndrome in children: Epidemiology, pathophysiology, diagnosis and sequelae. *Korean Journal of Pediatrics, 53*(10), 863-871. http://dx.doi.org/10.3345/kjp.2010.53.10.863.

Chang, A. M., Reid, K. J., Gourineni, R., & Zee, P. C. (2009). Sleep timing and circadian phase in delayed sleep phase syndrome. *Journal of Biological Rhythms, 24*(4), 313-321. http://dx.doi.org/10.1177/0748730409339611.

Chervin, R. D., Dillon, J. E., Archbold, K. H., & Ruzicka, D. L. (2003). Conduct problems and symptoms of sleep disorders in children. *Journal of the American Academy of Child & Adolescent Psychiatry, 42*(2), 201-208. https://doi.org/10.1097/00004583-200302000-00014.

Craske, M. G., & Tsao, J. C. (2005). Assessment and treatment of nocturnal panic attacks. *Sleep Medicine Reviews, 9*(3), 173-184. https://doi.org/10.1016/j.smrv.2004.11.003.

Dauvilliers, Y., Lopez, R., Ohayon, M., & Bayard, S. (2013). Hypersomnia and depressive symptoms: Methodological and clinical aspects. *BMC Medicine, 11*(1), 78. https://doi.org/10.1186/1741-7015-11-78.

Desai, A. V., Cherkas, L. F., Spector, T. D., & Williams, A. J. (2004). Genetic influences in self-reported symptoms of obstructive sleep apnea and restless legs: A twin study. *Twin Research & Human Genetics, 7*(6), 589-595. https://doi.org/10.1375/twin.7.6.589.

Dewald, J. F., Meijer, A. M., Oort, F. J., Kerkhof, G. A., & Bögels, S. M. (2010). The influence of sleep quality, sleep duration and sleepiness on school performance in children and adolescents: A meta-analytic review. *Sleep medicine reviews, 14*(3), 179-189. https://doi.org/10.1016/j.smrv.2009.10.004.

Dohnt, H., Gradisar, M., & Short, M. A. (2012). Insomnia and its symptoms in adolescents: Comparing DSM-IV and ICSD-II diagnostic criteria.

Journal of Clinical Sleep Medicine, 8(03), 295-299. http://dx.doi.org/10.5664/jcsm.1918.

Driver, H. S., & Shapiro, C. M. (1993). ABC of sleep disorders. Parasomnias. British Medical Journal, 306(6882), 921-924. https://doi.org/10.1136/bmj.306.6882.921.

Durmer, J. S., & Quraishi, G. H. (2011). Restless legs syndrome, periodic leg movements, and periodic limb movement disorder in children. Pediatric Clinics, 58(3), 591-620. https://doi.org/10.1016/j.pcl.2011.03.005.

Dye, T. J., Jain, S. V., & Kothare, S. V. (2015). Central hypersomnia. Seminars in pediatric neurology 22(2), 93-104. http://dx.doi.org/10.1016/j.spen.2015.03.004.

Einollahi, B., & Izadianmehr, N. (2014). Restless leg syndrome: A neglected diagnosis. Nephro-urology Monthly, 6(5), e22009. http://dx.doi.org/10.5812/numonthly.22009.

Fallone, G., Acebo, C., Seifer, R., & Carskadon, M. A. (2005). Experimental restriction of sleep opportunity in children: Effects on teacher ratings. Sleep, 28(12), 1561-1567. http://dx.doi.org/10.1093/sleep/28.12.1561.

Fallone, G., Owens, J. A., & Deane, J. (2002). Sleepiness in children and adolescents: Clinical implications. Sleep Medicine Reviews, 6(4), 287-306. https://doi.org/10.1053/smrv.2001.0192.

Faruqui, F., Khubchandani, J., Price, J. H., Bolyard, D., & Reddy, R. (2011). Sleep disorders in children: A national assessment of primary care pediatrician practices and perceptions. Pediatrics, 128(3), 539–546. https://doi.org/10.1542/peds.2011-0344.

Foral, P., Knezevich, J., Dewan, N., & Malesker, M. (2011). Medication-induced sleep disturbances. The Consultant Pharmacist, 26(6), 414-425. http://dx.doi.org/10.4140/TCP.n.2011.414.

Frucht, S., Rogers, J. D., Greene, P. E., Gordon, M. F., & Fahn, S. (1999). Falling asleep at the wheel: Motor vehicle mishaps in persons taking pramipexole and ropinirole. Neurology, 52(9), 1908. https://doi.org/10.1212/WNL.52.9.1908.

Gauchat, A., Séguin, J. R., & Zadra, A. (2014). Prevalence and correlates of disturbed dreaming in children. *Pathologie Biologie, 62*(5), 311-318. http://dx.doi.org/10.1016/j.patbio.2014.05.016.

Glozier, N., O'Dea, B., McGorry, P. D., Pantelis, C., Amminger, G. P., Hermens, D. F., Purcell, R., Scott, E., & Hickie, I. B. (2014). Delayed sleep onset in depressed young people. *BMC Psychiatry, 14*(1), 33-42. https://doi.org/10.1186/1471-244X-14-33.

Gradisar, M., & Crowley, S. J. (2013a). Delayed sleep phase disorder in youth. *Current Opinion in Psychiatry, 26*(6), 580-585. https://doi.org/10.1097/YCO.0b013e328365a1d4.

Gradisar, M., Wolfson, A. R., Harvey, A. G., Hale, L., Rosenberg, R., & Czeisler, C. A. (2013b). The sleep and technology use of Americans: Findings from the National Sleep Foundation's 2011 Sleep in America poll. *Journal of Clinical Sleep Medicine, 9*(12), 1291-1299. http://dx.doi.org/10.5664/jcsm.3272.

Gray, K. N., & Cromer, L. D. (2018). Posttraumatic nightmare content in children and its relation to posttraumatic psychopathology. *International Journal of Dream Research, 11*(2), 172-178. https://doi.org/10.11588/ijodr.2018.2.48777.

Groner, J. A., Nicholson, L., Huang, H., & Bauer, J. A. (2019). Secondhand smoke exposure and sleep-related breathing problems in toddlers. *Academic Pediatrics, 19*(7), 835-841. https://doi.org/10.1016/j.acap.2019.03.008.

Guilleminault, C., & Pelayo, R. (2000). Narcolepsy in children. *Pediatric Drugs, 2*(1), 1-9. https://doi.org/10.2165/00148581-200002010-00001.

Harvey, A. G. (2002). A cognitive model of insomnia. *Behaviour Research & Therapy, 40*(8), 869-893. https://doi.org/10.1016/S0005-7967(01)00061-4.

Hasler, B. P., Soehner, A. M., & Clark, D. B. (2014). Circadian rhythms and risk for substance use disorders in adolescence. *Current Opinion in Psychiatry, 27*(6), 460-466. http://dx.doi.org/10.1097/YCO.0000000000000107.

Hagenauer, M. H., Perryman, J. I., Lee, T. M., & Carskadon, M. A. (2009). Adolescent changes in the homeostatic and circadian regulation of sleep. *Developmental Neuroscience*, *31*(4), 276-284. doi: 10.1159/000216538.

Heussler, H. S. (2005). 9. Common causes of sleep disruption and daytime sleepiness: Childhood sleep disorders II. *Medical Journal of Australia*, *182*(9), 484-489. http://dx.doi.org/10.5694/j.1326-5377.2005.tb06793.x.

Hiller, R. M., Lovato, N., Gradisar, M., Oliver, M., & Slater, A. (2014). Trying to fall asleep while catastrophizing: What sleep-disordered adolescents think and feel. *Sleep Medicine*, *15*(1), 96-103. https://doi.org/10.1016/j.sleep.2013.09.014.

Honaker, S. M., & Meltzer, L. J. (2014). Bedtime problems and night wakings in young children: An update of the evidence. *Paediatric Respiratory Reviews*, *15*(4), 333–339. https://doi.org/10.1016/j.prrv.2014.04.011.

Hysing, M., Pallesen, S., Stormark, K. M., Lundervold, A. J., & Sivertsen, B. (2013). Sleep patterns and insomnia among adolescents: A population-based study. *Journal of Sleep Research*, *22*(5), 549-556. https://doi.org/10.1111/jsr.12055.

Högl, B., Kiechl, S., Willeit, J., Saletu, M., Frauscher, B., Seppi, K., Müller, J., Rungger, G., Gasperi, A., Wenning, G., & Poewe, W. (2005). Restless legs syndrome: A community-based study of prevalence, severity, and risk factors. *Neurology*, *64*(11), 1920–1924. https://doi.org/10.1212/01.WNL.0000163996.64461.A3.

Honaker, S. M., & Meltzer, L. J. (2016). Sleep in pediatric primary care: A review of the literature. *Sleep Medicine Reviews*, *25*, 31-39. https://doi.org/10.1016/j.smrv.2015.01.004.

Inocente, C. O., Gustin, M.-P., Lavault, S., Guignard-Perret, A., Raoux, A., Christol, N., Gerard, D., Dauvilliers, Y., Reimão, R., Bat-Pitault, F., Lin, J.-S., Arnulf, I., Lecendreux, M., & Franco, P. (2014). Quality of life in children with narcolepsy. *CNS Neuroscience & Therapeutics*, *20*(8), 763-771. https://doi.org/10.1111/cns.12291.

Irfan, M., Schenck, C. H., & Howell, M. J. (2017). Non–rapid eye movement sleep and overlap parasomnias. CONTINUUM: *Lifelong*

Learning in Neurology, 23(4), 1035-1050. https://doi.org/10.1212/CON.0000000000000503.

Johnson, E. O., & Roth, T. (2006). An epidemiologic study of sleep disordered breathing symptoms adolescents. *Sleep, 29*(9), 1135–1142. http://dx.doi.org/10.1093/sleep/29.9.1135.

Kaier, E., Zanotti, D., Davis, J. L., Strunk, K., & Cromer, L. D. (2016). Addressing the problem of student-athlete sleepiness: Feasibility of implementing an interactive sleep workshop at a Division I school. *Journal of Clinical Sport Psychology, 10*(3), 237-247.

Khan, Z., & Trotti, L. M. (2015). Central disorders of hypersomnolence. *Chest, 148*(1), 262-273. https://doi.org/10.1378/chest.14-1304.

Klackenberg, G. (1982). Somnambulism in childhood- prevalence, course and behavioral correlations: A prospective longitudinal study (6- 16 years). *Acta Paediatrica, 71*(3), 495-499. https://doi.org/10.1111/j.1651-2227.1982.tb09458.x.

Laberge, L., Petit, D., Simard, C., Vitaro, F., Tremblay, R. E., & Montplaisir, J. (2001). Development of sleep patterns in early adolescence. *Journal of Sleep Research, 10*(1), 59–67. https://doi.org/10.1046/j.1365-2869.2001.00242.x.

Langston, T. J., Davis, J. L., & Swopes, R. M. (2010). Idiopathic and posttrauma nightmares in a clinical sample of children and adolescents: Characteristics and related pathology. *Journal of Child & Adolescent Trauma, 3*(4), 344-356. https://doi.org/10.1080/19361521.2010.523064.

Lee, K. A., Mcenany, G., & Weekes, D. (1999). Gender differences in sleep patterns for early adolescents. *Journal of Adolescent Health, 24*(1), 16-20. https://doi.org/10.1016/S1054-139X(98)00074-3.

Lemyre, A., Bastien, C., & Vallières, A. (2019). Nightmares in mental disorders: A review. *Dreaming, 29*(2), 144-166. https://doi.org/10.1037/drm0000103.

Li, S. X., Yu, M. W. M., Lam, S. P., Zhang, J., Li, A. M., Lai, K. Y. C., & Wing, Y. K. (2011). Frequent nightmares in children: Familial aggregation and associations with parent-reported behavioral and mood problems. *Sleep, 34*(4), 487-493. https://doi.org/10.1093/sleep/34.4.487.

Lovato, N., Gradisar, M., Short, M., Dohnt, H., & Micic, G. (2013). Delayed sleep phase disorder in an Australian school-based sample of adolescents. *Journal of Clinical Sleep Medicine, 9*(09), 939-944. http://dx.doi.org/10.5664/jcsm.2998.

Lowenfeld, L. (1902). Ueber narkolepsie. *Muenchner Medizinische Wochenschrift, 49*, 1041–1045.

Lumeng, J. C., & Chervin, R. D. (2008). Epidemiology of pediatric obstructive sleep apnea. *Proceedings of the American Thoracic Society, 5*(2), 242-252. https://doi.org/10.1513/pats.200708-135MG.

Luo, R., Harding, R., Galland, B., Sellbom, M., Gill, A., & Schaughency, E. (2019). Relations between risk for sleep-disordered breathing, cognitive and executive functioning, and academic performance in six-year-olds. *Early Education & Development 30*(7), 947-970. https://doi.org/10.1080/10409289.2019.1593075.

Marcus, C. L. (2001). Sleep-disordered breathing in children. *American Journal of Respiratory & Critical Care Medicine, 164*(1), 16-30. http://dx.doi.org/10.1164/ajrccm.164.1.2008171.

Mason, T. B., & Pack, A. I. (2005). Sleep terrors in childhood. *The Journal of Pediatrics, 147*(3), 388-392. https://doi.org/10.1016/j.jpeds.2005.06.042.

Mason, T. B., & Pack, A. I. (2007). Pediatric parasomnias. *Sleep, 30*(2), 141-151. https://doi.org/10.1093/sleep/30.2.141.

Meltzer, L. J., Johnson, C., Crosette, J., Ramos, M., & Mindell, J. A. (2010). Prevalence of diagnosed sleep disorders in pediatric primary care practices. *Pediatrics, 125*(6), e1410-e1418. http://dx.doi.org/10.1542/peds.2009-2725.

Mignot, E. (1998). Genetic and familial aspects of narcolepsy. *Neurology, 50*(2 Suppl 1), S16-S22. http://dx.doi.org/10.1212/WNL.50.2_Suppl_1.S16.

Mindell, J. A., & Owens, J. A. (2015). *A clinical guide to pediatric sleep: Diagnosis and management of sleep problems* (3rd ed.). Wolters Kluwer.

Montplaisir, J., Boucher, S., Poirier, G., Lavigne, G., Lapierre, O., & Lespérance, P. (1997). Clinical, polysomnographic, and genetic characteristics of restless legs syndrome: A study of 133 patients diagnosed with new standard criteria. *Movement Disorders: Official Journal of the Movement Disorder Society, 12*(1), 61-65. https://doi.org/10.1002/mds.870120111.

Muris, P., Merckelbach, H., Ollendick, T. H., King, N. J., & Bogie, N. (2001). Children's nighttime fears: Parent–child ratings of frequency, content, origins, coping behaviors and severity. *Behaviour Research & Therapy, 39*(1), 13-28. http://dx.doi.org/10.1016/S0005-7967(99)00155-2.

Natarajan, N., Jain, S. V., Chaudhry, H., Hallinan, B. E., & Simakajornboon, N. (2013). Narcolepsy-cataplexy: Is streptococcal infection a trigger? *Journal of Clinical Sleep Medicine, 9*(03), 269-270. http://dx.doi.org/10.5664/jcsm.2498.

Narayanan, A., Yogesh, A., Mitchell, R. B., & Johnson, R. F. (2019). Asthma and obesity as predictors of severe obstructive sleep apnea in an adolescent pediatric population. *The Laryngoscope. 160*(1), 150-157. https://doi.org/10.1002/lary.28029.

Nesbitt, A. D. (2018). Delayed sleep-wake phase disorder. *Journal of Thoracic Disease, 10*(Suppl 1), 103-111. http://dx.doi.org/10.21037/jtd.2018.01.11.

Nevsimalova, S. (2014). The diagnosis and treatment of pediatric narcolepsy. *Current Neurology & Neuroscience Reports, 14*(8), 469. https://doi.org/10.1007/s11910-014-0469-1.

Nguyen, B. H., Pérusse, D., Paquet, J., Petit, D., Boivin, M., Tremblay, R. E., & Montplaisir, J. (2008). Sleep terrors in children: A prospective study of twins. *Pediatrics, 122*(6), 1164-1167. http://dx.doi.org/10.1542/peds.2008-1303.

Ohayon, M. M., Priest, R. G., Zulley, J., Smirne, S., & Paiva, T. (2002). Prevalence of narcolepsy symptomatology and diagnosis in the European general population. *Neurology, 58*(12), 1826-1833. https://doi.org/10.1212/wnl.58.12.1826.

Ohayon, M. M., Roberts, R. E., Zulley, J., Smirne, S., & Priest, R. G. (2000). Prevalence and patterns of problematic sleep among older adolescents. *Journal of the American Academy of Child & Adolescent Psychiatry, 39*(12), 1549-1556. https://doi.org/10.1097/00004583-200012000-00019.

Owens, J. A. (2001). The practice of pediatric sleep medicine: Results of a community survey. *Pediatrics, 108*(3), e51. https://doi.org/10.1542/peds.108.3.e51.

Owens, J. A. (2005). Epidemiology of sleep disorders during childhood. In S. H. Heldon, R. Ferber, & M. H. Kryger (Eds.), *Principles & practice of pediatric sleep medicine* (pp. 27-33). WB Saunders. http://dx.doi.org/10.1016/B978-0-7216-9458-0.50008-8.

Owens, J. A. (2019). Behavioral sleep problems in children. In A. G. Hoppin (Ed.), *UpToDate*. Retrieved June 23, 2019, from https://www.uptodate.com/contents/behavioral-sleep-problems-in-children.

Owens, J. A., & Mindell, J. A. (2011). Pediatric insomnia. *Pediatric Clinics, 58*(3), 555-569. https://doi.org/10.1016/j.pcl.2011.03.011.

Owens, J., Spirito, A., Nobile, C., & Arrigan, M. (1997). Incidence of parasomnias in children with obstructive sleep apnea. *Sleep, 20*(12), 1193-1196. https://doi.org/10.1093/sleep/20.12.1193.

Picchietti, D., Allen, R. P., Walters, A. S., Davidson, J. E., Myers, A., & Ferini-Strambi, L. (2007). Restless legs syndrome: Prevalence and impact in children and adolescents—the Peds REST study. *Pediatrics, 120*(2), 253-266. https://doi.org/10.1542/peds.2006-2767.

Picchietti, D. L., Arbuckle, R. A., Abetz, L., Durmer, J. S., Ivanenko, A., Owens, J. A., & Walters, A. S. (2011). Pediatric restless legs syndrome: Analysis of symptom descriptions and drawings. *Journal of Child Neurology, 26*(11), 1365-1376. doi: 10.1177/0883073811 405852.

Picchietti, D. L., Bruni, O., de Weerd, A., Durmer, J. S., Kotagal, S., Owens, J. A., & Simakajornboon, N. (2013). Pediatric restless legs syndrome diagnostic criteria: An update by the International Restless Legs

Syndrome Study Group. *Sleep Medicine, 14*(12), 1253–1259. https://doi.org/10.1016/j.sleep.2013.08.778.

Punamäki, R. L., Ali, K. J., Ismahil, K. H., & Nuutinen, J. (2005). Trauma, dreaming, and psychological distress among Kurdish children. *Dreaming, 15*(3), 178-194. https://doi.org/10.1037/1053-0797.15.3.178.

Reynolds, K. C., & Alfano, C. A. (2015). Things that go bump in the night: Frequency and predictors of nightmares in anxious and nonanxious children. *Behavioral Sleep Medicine, 14*(4), 442-456. http://dx.doi.org/10.1080/15402002.2015.1017099.

Richardson, M., & Friedman, N. (Eds.). (2016). *Clinician's Guide to Pediatric Sleep Disorders.* CRC Press.

Rodriguez, A. J. (2007). Pediatric sleep and epilepsy. *Current Neurology & Neuroscience Reports, 7*(4), 342-347. https://doi.org/10.1007/s11910-007-0052-0.

Rosen, R. C., Zozula, R., Jahn, E. G., & Carson, J. L. (2001). Low rates of recognition of sleep disorders in primary care: Comparison of a community-based versus clinical academic setting. *Sleep Medicine, 2*(1), 47-55. http://dx.doi.org/10.1016/S1389-9457(00)00043-5.

Sánchez-Armengol, A., Ruiz-García, A., Carmona-Bernal, C., Botebol-Benhamou, G., García-Díaz, E., Polo-Padillo, J., López-Campos, J. L., & Capote, F. (2008). Clinical and polygraphic evolution of sleep-related breathing disorders in adolescents. *European Respiratory Journal, 32*(4), 1016–1022. https://doi.org/10.1183/09031936.00133907.

Saxvig, I. W., Pallesen, S., Wilhelmsen-Langeland, A., Molde, H., & Bjorvatn, B. (2012). Prevalence and correlates of delayed sleep phase in high school students. *Sleep Medicine, 13*(2), 193-199. https://doi.org/10.1016/j.sleep.2011.10.024.

Scherrer, V., Roberts, R., & Preckel, F. (2016). Parents' assessment of circadian preference in elementary school-aged children: Validity and relations to educational outcomes. *Chronobiology International, 33*(9), 1188-1207. https://doi.org/10.1080/07420528.2016.1210618.

Schredl, M., Fricke-Oerkermann, L., Mitschke, A., Wiater, A., & Lehmkuhl, G. (2009a). Factors affecting nightmares in children: Parents' vs. children's ratings. *European Child & Adolescent Psychiatry, 18*(1), 20-25. https://doi.org/10.1007/s00787-008-0697-5.

Schredl, M., Fricke-Oerkermann, L., Mitschke, A., Wiater, A., & Lehmkuhl, G. (2009b). Longitudinal study of nightmares in children: Stability and effect of emotional symptoms. *Child Psychiatry & Human Development, 40*(3), 439-449. https://doi.org/10.1007/s10578-009-0136-y.

Secrist, M. E., Dalenberg, C. J., & Gevirtz, R. (2019). Contributing factors predicting nightmares in children: Trauma, anxiety, dissociation, and emotion regulation. *Psychological Trauma: Theory, Research, Practice, & Policy, 11*(1), 114-121. https://doi.org/10.1037/tra0000387.

Sedky, K., Bennett, D. S., & Carvalho, K. S. (2014). Attention deficit hyperactivity disorder and sleep disordered breathing in pediatric populations: A meta-analysis. *Sleep Medicine Reviews, 18*(4), 349-356. https://doi.org/10.1016/j.smrv.2013.12.003.

Silber, M. H., Krahn, L. E., Olson, E. J., & Pankratz, V. S. (2002). The epidemiology of narcolepsy in Olmsted County, Minnesota: A population-based study. *Sleep, 25*(2), 197–202. https://doi.org/10.1093/sleep/25.2.197.

Spilsbury, J. C., Storfer-Isser, A., Kirchner, H. L., Nelson, L., Rosen, C. L., Drotar, D., & Redline, S. (2006). Neighborhood disadvantage as a risk factor for pediatric obstructive sleep apnea. *The Journal of Pediatrics, 149*(3), 342-347. https://doi.org/10.1016/j.jpeds.2006.04.061.

Stores, G. (2007). Parasomnias of childhood and adolescence. *Sleep Medicine Clinics, 2*(3), 405-417. http://dx.doi.org/10.1016/j.jsmc.2007.05.014.

Stores, G., Montgomery, P., & Wiggs, L. (2006). The psychosocial problems of children with narcolepsy and those with excessive daytime sleepiness of uncertain origin. *Pediatrics, 118*(4), e1116-e1123. https://doi.org/10.1542/peds.2006-0647.

Talih, F. R. (2011). Narcolepsy presenting as schizophrenia: A literature review and two case reports. *Innovations in Clinical Neuroscience, 8*(4), 30-34.

Thiedke, C. C. (2001). Sleep disorders and sleep problems in childhood. *American Family Physician, 63*(2), 277-284.

Thomas, J. H., & Burgers, D. E. (2018). Sleep is an eye-opener: Behavioral causes and consequences of hypersomnolence in children. *Paediatric Respiratory Reviews, 25*, 3-8. https://doi.org/10.1016/j.prrv.2016.11.004.

Valli, K., Revonsuo, A., Pälkäs, O., & Punamäki, R. L. (2006). The effect of trauma on dream content--A field study of Palestinian children. *Dreaming, 16*(2), 63-87. https://doi.org/10.1037/1053-0797.16.2.63.

Vriend, J., & Corkum, P. (2011). Clinical management of behavioral insomnia of childhood. *Psychology research & behavior management, 4*, 69. https://dx.doi.org/10.2147%2FPRBM.S14057.

Walters, A. S., Hickey, K., Maltzman, J., Verrico, T., Joseph, D., Hening, W., Wilson, V., & Chokroverty, S. (1996). A questionnaire study of 138 patients with restless legs syndrome: The Night-Walkers' survey. *Neurology, 46* (1), 92-95. https://doi.org/10.1212/wnl.46.1.92.

Watson, L. A., Phillips, A. J., Hosken, I. T., McGlashan, E. M., Anderson, C., Lack, L. C., Lockley, S. W., Rajaratnam, S. M. W., & Cain, S. W. (2018). Increased sensitivity of the circadian system to light in delayed sleep–wake phase disorder. *The Journal of Physiology, 596*(24), 6249-6261. https://doi.org/10.1113/JP275917.

Weintraub, Y., Singer, S., Alexander, D., Hacham, S., Menuchin, G., Lubetzky, R., Steinberg, D. M., & Pinhas-Hamiel, O. (2013). Enuresis—an unattended comorbidity of childhood obesity. *International Journal of Obesity, 37*(1), 75-78. https://doi.org/10.1038/ijo.2012.108.

Wickersham, L. (2006). Time-of-day preference for preschool-aged children. *Chrestomathy: Annual Review of Undergraduate Research, 5*, 259-268.

Yoon, S. Y. R., Jain, U., & Shapiro, C. (2012). Sleep in attention-deficit/hyperactivity disorder in children and adults: Past, present, and future. *Sleep Medicine Reviews, 16*(4), 371-388. http://dx.doi.org/10.1016/j.smrv.2011.07.001.

Zucconi, M., & Ferini-Strambi, L. (2000). NREM parasomnias: arousal disorders and differentiation from nocturnal frontal lobe epilepsy. *Clinical Neurophysiology, 111*(Suppl. 2), S129-S135. https://doi.org/10.1016/S1388-2457(00)00413-2.

Zucconi, M., & Ferini-Strambi, L. (2004). Epidemiology and clinical findings of restless legs syndrome. *Sleep Medicine, 5*(3), 293-299. https://doi.org/10.1016/j.sleep.2004.01.004.

In: Children and Sleep
Editor: Olivie Gadbois

ISBN: 978-1-53618-074-9
© 2020 Nova Science Publishers, Inc.

Chapter 3

THE IMPORTANCE OF SLEEP ON CHILDHOOD NEURODEVELOPMENT

Negin Badihian and Roya Kelishadi[*]

Child Growth and Development Research Center, Research Institute for Primordial Prevention of Non-Communicable Disease, Isfahan University of Medical Sciences, Isfahan, Iran

ABSTRACT

Sleep is an essential time and process in human life. We spend almost one third of our life sleeping or trying to fall asleep. It is especially important when it comes to minors; about forty percent of the childhood period is spent in sleep. Intense brain activities that involve higher cortical functions and significant physiological activities occur during sleep. Therefore, it led some scientists to conclude that brain is more active during sleep compared to the wakeful state. Sleep is considered to have influential roles in neural plasticity, brain development, and skill learning during childhood. Moreover, it would affect capability of acquiring new skills and exploring the environment when facing a new situation. It is reported that one third of children experience some degrees of sleep disturbances. The circadian and homeostatic systems are both responsible for sleep

---

[*] Corresponding Author's Email: roya.kelishadi@gmail.com, and Kelishadi@med.mui.ac.ir.

regulation. Sleep duration, quality, timing, regularity, and absence of sleep disturbances are all important for the proper function of brain and body. The adequate duration of sleep varies between individuals; it is influenced by the complex interactions of genetic and environmental factors. But in general, the required duration of sleep is much longer in newborns, i.e., 12-16 hours a day, and has a gradual decrease to 8-10 hours a day in teenagers. The proportion of rapid eye movement (REM) and non-REM sleeps are also affected by age because of the different functions of these states. While newborns have equal REM and non-REM duration, REM sleep would gradually decrease as the child grows up. Sleep problems diminish normal brain function and would result in short- and long-term adverse health effects. Inadequate sleep duration or quality during childhood might cause dysfunctions in the attention, behavior, cognition, and working memory, which in turn would cause hyperactivity and poor impulse control, decreased intellectual ability, and learning problems. It would further increase the risk of hypertension, obesity, diabetes, and other psychological problems including depression. However, increased duration of daily sleep would also result in hypertension, diabetes, obesity and psychological disorders. Additionally, sleep disturbances can affect high level cognitive functions (e.g., abstract thinking and cognitive flexibility) and even might affect brain morphology in distinct regions. In this chapter, we aim to summarize the importance of healthy sleep cycle in normal brain development during childhood and the effects of sleep disturbances on normal brain function and brain structure.

INTRODUCTION

Nearly, all organisms, including insects and worms, sleep (Zielinski, McKenna, and McCarley 2016). Sleep is essential in human life and is known to affect all systems in the body. Some of the important body organs and functions affected by sleep are cardiovascular system, body metabolism, immune system, endocrine system, mental health, and development (Paruthi et al. 2016). Considering the critical role of sleep in brain and body homeostasis, any dysregulation can cause adverse health consequences (Zielinski, McKenna, and McCarley 2016). For instance, studies have shown the association between inadequate sleep and attention deficits, behavioral problems, learning difficulties, increased risk of accidents, cardiovascular diseases (e.g., hypertension), metabolic syndrome, obesity, diabetes, and mental health issues. On the other hand, oversleeping may also cause such complications (Paruthi et al. 2016). Sleep is especially important for children and adolescents considering the important role it plays in brain maturation and development. By the age of 3, the child has spent most of their life asleep and by the age of 18, 40% of an individual's life has been spent sleeping (El Shakankiry 2011, Meltzer 2017). During childhood, the developing brain has its highest plasticity and maximum capacity to learn tasks and acquire skills in response to various stimuli; the brain undergoes fundamental changes in this period of age (Wilhelm, Diekelmann, and Born 2008). Scientists suggest that standard sleep is critical for these processes, as sleep disorders during childhood may lead to persistent significant adverse outcomes in different areas of neurodevelopment (Fischer, Wilhelm, and Born 2007). From an epidemiologic point of view, approximately one third of all children and 25% of those aged <5 years show some types of sleep disorders (El Shakankiry 2011). Also, in a community sample of children aged 4 to 10 years the prevalence of sleep disorders was reported to be 37%. Similarly, the prevalence of sleep disorders remain high in adolescence with 40% of the adolescents reporting some degrees of sleep problems (El Shakankiry 2011). Hence, it is of great importance to appreciate the effects of sleep disorders on children and adolescents and implement efficacious studies to address the issue and prevent unfavorable consequences.

In the present chapter, we would first describe the characteristics of standard sleep, the underlying mechanisms responsible for sleep regulation during childhood and adolescence, and the importance of sleep for brain maturation and development. Then we would discuss the effects of sleep disorders on neurodevelopment from both basic and clinical aspects.

NORMAL SLEEP CYCLE IN CHILDHOOD AND THE EFFECTS OF SLEEP ON NEURODEVELOPMENT

Sleep physiology is very complex. Various cellular and molecular mechanisms are involved in sleep initiation, regulation, and maintenance (Eban-Rothschild, Appelbaum, and de Lecea 2018). Generally, gross physiologic presentations of sleep are the first signs to determine the meaning of sleep. These gross presentations also vary between non-rapid eye movement (NREM) and REM sleep cycles (El Shakankiry 2011). NREM sleep physiologic presentations include increased muscle blood flow, low postural muscle tone, decreased eye movements, slow rhythmic breathing, decreased heart rate, restoration of energy, repairment of tissues, and secretion of hormones essential for growth and development (Maski and Owens 2016, Zielinski, McKenna, and McCarley 2016). REM sleep is determined by dreaming, facial expressions, dialogues and vocalizations related to the dream, twitching of muscles, complete loss of muscle tone in the axial postural muscles (REM paralysis), and irregular breathing and heart rate (Logan et al. 2018, El Shakankiry 2011). In newborns, minimal muscle movements and cycles of rhythmic breathing are the main gross changes during quiet sleep, which is parallel to NREM sleep. Sucking gestures, twitches, both smiling and frowning, limb movements, and irregular breathing happen during active sleep of newborns, which is equivalent to REM sleep (El Shakankiry 2011).

Intense brain activities that involve higher cortical functions and significant physiological events occur during sleep (El Shakankiry 2011, Kurth et al. 2015). Brain physiologic changes during sleep in human are mainly recognized using electroencephalogram (EEG) recordings (Kurth et al. 2013, Rusterholz et al. 2018). These EEG signals include brain wave fluctuations such as presence of delta frequency, also called slow wave, during NREM sleep. Other EEG waves seen during NREM sleep are sleep spindles and some special patterns (e.g., K-complexes). In contrary, REM sleep is identified with theta and gamma waves (Zielinski, McKenna, and McCarley 2016). These brain wave alterations are the results of ionic current changes in the neurons and glial cells (Zielinski, McKenna, and McCarley 2016). The proportion of sleep associated with specific wave patterns undergoes changes as the child grows up and is affected by age. For instance, during childhood, slow wave sleep is greater than adulthood (Wilhelm, Diekelmann, and Born 2008). These brain EEG frequencies can give us valuable information on the brain health. Consequently, sleep EEG has been suggested as an important tool to detect sleep problems (Kurth et al. 2013,

Chu et al. 2014). Delta wave power density is reported to differ between newborns with normal birth weights and those small for gestational age. Delta wave power is also higher in healthy term newborns compared to preterm babies (Shellhaas et al. 2017). Moreover, sleep EEG can provide valuable information on the psychologic and behavioral problems in children. For example, slow wave activity (EEG activities of 1-4.5 Hz) is highly sensitive for investigating maturational differences in experience-dependent plasticity (Wilhelm et al. 2014). Sleep spindles (transient 10-16 Hz oscillations with a duration of 0.5-2 s) are cortical activities that reflect inter-regional brain communications during NREM sleep and the maturational status of thalamocortical pathways (Gomez and Edgin 2015, Bódizs et al. 2014). These brain EEG activities are associated with memory consolidation, social skills development, intelligence quotient (IQ), learning skills, and improved retention of new skills in preschool children and adults. Therefore, reduced sleep spindles could be seen in some medical conditions such as intellectual disabilities (Brockmann et al. 2019, Rusterholz et al. 2018, Bódizs et al. 2014). During adolescence, amplitude and power of sleep EEG significantly decrease. This decline is driven by the considerable reduction of cortical gray matter that normally occurs throughout adolescence. It usually happens in girls earlier than boys and is linked to puberty (Logan et al. 2018, Tarokh, Saletin, and Carskadon 2016).

From the cellular perspective, there are evidences that suggest sleep is regulated through the same cellular pathways that inflammation and neurotransmission are modulated (Zielinski, McKenna, and McCarley 2016). Hypothalamic neurons regulate sleep by suppressing the arousal system. Sleep-wake cycle, which determines sleep and wakefulness, is regulated by light and dark cycle through circadian rhythm and homeostatic process. Homeostatic regulation of sleep happens in response to the duration of wakefulness. As the duration of wakefulness period increases, the drive to sleep increases proportionately (Barone, Hawks-Mayer, and Lipton 2019). The development of sleep-wake cycle requires time; Hence, newborns show an irregular sleep pattern. The sleep-wake cycle starts to develop around 2 months of age; by 6 months of age, the rhythm would have an almost regular pattern with cyclic phases of NREM and REM sleep, which are also the hallmarks of adult sleep (Gomez and Edgin 2015). By 6-9 months of age, most of the infants could sleep throughout the night without any need for a nighttime feeding (Mindell et al. 2017). Neurons of the pons send outputs to different brain and spinal cord regions to shift between NREM and REM sleep throughout the night sleep (Tashjian, Goldenberg, and Galvan 2017). Scientists suggest that stages 3 and 4 of NREM sleep are the most restorative phases of sleep, while REM sleep is known to be the learning time from the day experiences (Medic, Wille, and Hemels 2017). So, it seems reasonable to have more proportion of REM sleep during infancy, as high as 55%. This proportion decreases as the child grows up and reaches almost 20-25% by the age of 5 (El Shakankiry 2011).

It is suggested that sleep-wake rhythm variability is highest during adolescence (Dahl and Lewin 2002). Various physiologic, social and environmental factors could affect the circadian rhythm, the daily rhythm of physiology, and behavior in this age period. These factors include gender, body temperature, noise, usual mealtime, physical activity, bedtime routines, presence of pain, and used medications (El Shakankiry 2011, Medic, Wille, and Hemels 2017). Moreover, immune system activity, brain development, and cognition are some of the other physiologic factors that could influence the brain regions and networks responsible for the regulation of vigilance state and play roles in the regulation of sleep phases (Zielinski, McKenna, and McCarley 2016). Moreover, the circadian rhythm controls metabolism, basal body temperature, heart rate, muscle tone, and endocrine secretions (Medic, Wille, and Hemels 2017). It is suggested that children would show a preference of circadian sleep rhythm by the age of 6. However, as the child grows up, they would encounter more challenges to have a normal regular sleep (El Shakankiry 2011). Another important component of circadian rhythm is the neurohormone melatonin. The suprachiasmatic nucleus is directly connected to the retinal nerve cells that detect brightness as the major stimulus. The suprachiasmatic nucleus sends a message to the pineal gland for melatonin secretion. Eventually, the circadian rhythm synchronize sleep with the 24 hours day-night cycle and the body homeostasis through melatonin (Medic, Wille, and Hemels 2017).

These mechanisms, if all work normally, ultimately let the child experience the standard sleep. A standard sleep is recognized by adequate duration, good quality, proper regularity and appropriate timing without any kind of sleep related problems (Medic, Wille, and Hemels 2017).

The amount of sleep needed for a normal and healthy development decreases by growing up. The normal range of sleep widely differs between infants under 4 months of age but would reach an almost stable range later. The needed sleep is assumed to be as follows: by 4 to 12 months of age, 12-16 hours/day; by 1-2 years of age, 11 to 14 hours/day; and by 3 to 5 years of age, 10 -13 hours/day (Willumsen and Bull 2020). These sleep durations include both nighttime sleep and daily naps. Although napping is common among children under 3 years old, it would be usually discontinued by the ages 3 to 5 years (Institute of Medicine Committee on Sleep and Research 2006). In pre-school children 9-12 hours/day of sleep are needed, and this amount would decrease to 8-10 h/d by adolescence (Paruthi et al. 2016). Age is the primary determinant of how much sleep is needed. However, medical conditions, gender, genetics, biological status, psychosocial factors, lifestyle, geography, culture, and environment could also affect normal sleep pattern and duration through the mechanisms stated above. Hence, even in a specific age range there could be different sleeping behaviors between individuals (Paruthi et al. 2016, Medic, Wille, and Hemels 2017, Zhao, Zhao, and Veasey 2017).

Brain development is speculated to be the main goal of sleep (Telzer et al. 2015). It is suggested that the newborn's sleep reflects the integrity of brain function (Shellhaas et al. 2017). Results of a study on kittens showed enhanced cortical plasticity during the important period of visual development in sleep and not wakefulness (Frank, Issa, and Stryker 2001). Usually, enough sleeping would lead to an enhanced attention, memory consolidation, improved learning, emotional stabilization and better behavioral, mental, and physical health. It is also positively associated with cognitive performance in children (Philbrook et al. 2017, Telzer et al. 2015). Studies have shown that children with better sleep qualities show better performance on various neurobehavioral tasks, especially tasks related to working memory and crystalized intelligence (Philbrook et al. 2017). Some investigators have suggested that neural networks involved in sleep dependent memory formation change fundamentally from infancy to early childhood (Gomez and Edgin 2015). Sleep facilitates generalization in infants and enhances the precise memory after the child reaches 18-24 months of age (Gomez and Edgin 2015). Sleep is also indicated to affect the general IQ. Previous studies have reported positive correlations between IQ and the magnitude of sleep spindles (i.e., power, amplitude and density) in both children and adolescents (Tarokh, Saletin, and Carskadon 2016, Bodizs et al. 2014). A study conducted on low birth weight premature infants showed that sleep organization (defined based on the sleep-state transitions) was associated with the status of executive functioning and verbal IQ by the age of 5 years (Weisman et al. 2011). Moreover, during brain activity and wakefulness, some molecular wastes such as reactive oxygen species are produced by neural cells. These noxious substances are potentially damaging for the brain cells and should be cleared through perivascular channels. Investigations have shown an increased clearance of these metabolic substances during sleep compared to wakefulness (Zielinski, McKenna, and McCarley 2016).

Sleep is known to affect the brain morphology and myelin maturation. Results from a study supported the hypothesis on the important role of sleep on myelin maturation during childhood. Using sleep EEG, the investigators showed that the frontal/occipital slow wave activity (F/O-ratio) during childhood can significantly predict the whole brain myelin of 3.5 years later (LeBourgeois et al. 2019). In another study, sleep duration was positively correlated with the gray matter volume of bilateral hippocampus in children and adolescents 5 to 18 years old (Taki et al. 2012). Another study found an association between sleep variability in adolescents and white matter integrity (Telzer et al. 2015).

Scientists speculate that there are many other aspects of brain maturation and development in children and adolescents that may get affected by sleep and currently we barely know about them (Meltzer 2017). In the rest of this chapter, we would explain some of the deficits and adverse effects caused by sleep disorders during childhood.

THE EFFECTS OF CHILDHOOD SLEEP DISTURBANCES ON THE BRAIN

Childhood sleep problems are the fifth leading cause of concern for parents (El Shakankiry 2011). Studies have shown that these problems are more serious concerns for parents compared to some other important issues such as language and motor development difficulties or toileting (Mindell and Owens 2003).Several studies assessing the prevalence of sleep problems in preschool children reported the overall prevalence of 25 to 50% (El Shakankiry 2011). A study in United States reported that 97% of the 12th grade students had inadequate sleep duration per night when compared to the recommended sleep duration for their age (Institute of Medicine Committee on Sleep and Research 2006, Zhao, Zhao, and Veasey 2017). Some neurodevelopmental conditions such as autism and developmental delays significantly affect the prevalence and severity of sleep problems in children. For instance, the prevalence of sleep disorders in autistic children are reported to be as high as 80% (Meltzer 2017). Sleep disorders generally present with inadequate sleep duration, low quality sleep, difficulty in maintaining sleep, or sleep-related problems, such as sleep apnea (Medic, Wille, and Hemels 2017).

Studies using animals and human adults showed altered synaptic plasticity following sleep disturbances like sleep deprivation (Jan et al. 2010). Alterations in the synaptic plasticity would further lead to transcriptional changes related to protein synthesis, decreased volume of brain gray matter in cortical and subcortical regions, and reduced brain metabolism (Telzer et al. 2015). Studies on adult animals also reported increased expression of genes involved in stress responses, like proteasomal pathways and chaperones, following inadequate sleep (Barone, Hawks-Mayer, and Lipton 2019). Abnormal sleep leads to the expression of genes that could cause cellular growth arrest and ultimately impair neurodevelopment (Kocevska et al. 2016). Sleep disturbances are linked to disturbed neuroplasticity, increased activity of the sympathetic nervous system, augmented hypothalamic-pituitary-adrenal axis activity, increased serum level of corticosterone, proinflammatory responses, and changes in the metabolism (Medic, Wille, and Hemels 2017, Telzer et al. 2015). A study that evaluated the short- and long-term health consequences of sleep disturbances suggested that the underlying mechanisms of these consequences are similar. They reported that the duration of sleep disturbance would determine the outcome (Medic, Wille, and Hemels 2017).

Sleep deprivation can result in reduced brain volume, neural death, and increased risk of further emotional and behavioral problems during critical period of development (Zielinski, McKenna, and McCarley 2016). Neurocognitive consequences following sleep disorders are reported in older infants and children (Shellhaas et al. 2017). Also, there are evidences that frequent snoring is significantly associated with lower cognitive scores in medically healthy infants (Shellhaas et al. 2017). Based on EEG recordings of youth, poor sleep significantly affects neural functioning and would cause memory formation impairment, learning problems, difficulties with executive functioning, and psychological wellbeing impairments (Jan et al. 2010). Evidently, sleep disorders in children and adolescents could affect all aspects of functioning and generally present with sleepiness besides other consequences (Philbrook et al. 2017, Kurth et al. 2015). Sleepiness in children and adolescents may not present with the classic signs of sleepiness that occur in adults. Sleepiness in children and adolescents usually manifest by mood and behavioral instabilities and neurocognitive dysfunctions, such as hyperactivity, impulsive behaviors, and attention deficits. Sleep problems would also lead to the impairments in learning, cognitive flexibility, abstract thinking, reasoning, and memory in children (El Shakankiry 2011, Maski and Owens 2016). Studies have reported a bidirectional association between somatic complaints and sleep disturbances in adolescents which may be due to the common underlying risk factors both disorders have (Medic, Wille, and Hemels 2017). The severity of common gastrointestinal disorders, especially functional gastrointestinal disorders, increases following sleep problems (Tarokh, Saletin, and Carskadon 2016). Studies have reported that the quality of life of children and adolescents decreases significantly following sleep disorders, especially in those suffering an underlying neurodevelopmental disability such as autism (Angriman et al. 2015).

Authors of a study suggested that the coincidence maturation of sleep mechanisms with synaptic plasticity is among the main reasons responsible for the presence of sleep disturbances in children suffering neurodevelopmental disorders (Barone, Hawks-Mayer, and Lipton 2019). While normally developing children experience some transient age-related changes in their sleep pattern (for example during puberty), sleep disturbances in children diagnosed with neurodevelopmental disabilities are usually chronic and continue to adolescence and even adulthood (Angriman et al. 2015, Barone, Hawks-Mayer, and Lipton 2019). Sleep disturbances can worsen the condition of a child suffering neurodevelopmental disabilities bring additional learning and behavioral problems and affect the family's quality of life (D'Souza et al. 2019). These children mainly complain of night settling difficulties and nocturnal awakening. The insomnia in these patients is chronic and with a prevalence much greater than normally developing children (Barone, Hawks-Mayer, and Lipton 2019). Sleep also plays roles in the underlying neural networks and mechanisms important for memory formation. Inadequate sleep impairs creation of long-term task related memories following consolidation of learned skills (Barone, Hawks-Mayer, and Lipton 2019). Sleep disturbances also affect psychosocial behaviors significantly (Philbrook et al. 2017). It is reported that poor sleep quality is associated with higher affect-related impulsivity but not response inhibition and cognitive impulsivity among adolescents (Tashjian, Goldenberg, and Galvan 2017). A systematic review of 76 studies on adolescents showed that sleep deprivation is significantly associated with negative consequences in many health aspects, primarily psychosocial and somatic health, school performance and the probability of having risky behaviors (Shochat, Cohen-Zion, and Tzischinsky 2014). Nicotine and marijuana abuse were among the most important risky behaviors associated with sleep loss as reported by this systematic review (Shochat, Cohen-Zion, and Tzischinsky 2014). Inadequate sleep among US high school students was reported to be associated with an increased risk of self-harm, tendency to suicide (suicidal thoughts and attempts), driving while being drunk, carrying weapon, smoking, drinking alcohol, using marijuana, risky sexual behaviors, and texting while driving (Tarokh,

Saletin, and Carskadon 2016). The relationship between unhealthy sleep pattern and diminished school performance is reported in several studies. A study conducted on adolescents reported earlier bedtime, longer sleep duration through weekdays, and less daytime sleepiness in those with better school performance compared to students with poorer school performance (Medic, Wille, and Hemels 2017).

Although immediate effects of neural changing from sleep disturbances may not be detectable, chronic sleep problems would have an accumulating effect and can impair neural integrity, decrease the level of neurogenesis, and alter structural plasticity, progressively (Telzer et al. 2015). Chronic sleep loss significantly affects neural mechanisms related to synaptic plasticity and is accompanied with poorer developmental outcomes and behavioral problems (Barone, Hawks-Mayer, and Lipton 2019). A study conducted in China on children aged 5 to 12 years reported a mean prevalence of 9.8% for chronic sleep disturbances with higher prevalence among boys (Li et al. 2014). Chronic sleep deprivation and circadian disruptions affect brain development processes and increase the chance of presenting risky behaviors, including substance abuse engagement, through increasing the sensitivity of reward circuit and impulsivity in adolescents (Logan et al. 2018).

Studies suggest that sleep disorders, especially during brain development, may have persistent health consequences which continue in future (Zhao, Zhao, and Veasey 2017). Based on the results from experimental studies, persistent neuronal damage and loss of some types of neurons occur following chronic inadequate sleep with long-term effects on sleep-wake cycles (Zhao, Zhao, and Veasey 2017). Findings from a study conducted on Drosophila melanogaster highlighted the importance of adequate sleep during brain development period (Seugnet et al. 2011). When flies underwent sleep loss at the first day beyond the larva stage, they represented memory impairments lasting for at least 6 days. However, in adult flies experiencing equal amount of sleep loss, although some degrees of learning deficits were presented, the effects were disappeared by few hours of compensatory sleep (Seugnet et al. 2011). Another study on Drosophila flies also indicated the importance of adequate sleep during critical period of brain development for normal courtship behaviors later in adulthood (Kayser, Yue, and Sehgal 2014). Abnormal courtship behaviors were accompanied with developmental impairments of a specific olfactory glomerulus. This study suggested that the most vulnerable brain regions to sleep disturbances during early life were regions with the highest growing velocity (Kayser, Yue, and Sehgal 2014). Results from a human cohort study indicated that although sleep disturbances during infancy and under 2 years of age were not related to the brain morphology at 7 years of age, such disturbances after 2 years of age were significantly associated with decreased gray matter volume at the age of 7 years. Also, the reduced prefrontal cortex volume was observed in these children (Kocevska et al. 2016). Moreover, higher quiet sleep proportion, known by sleep EEG, in healthy term neonates was reported to be significantly associated with decreased motor development by 6 months of age (Shellhaas et al. 2017). It is indicated that inefficient neonatal sleep can predict adverse long-term outcomes in babies suffering neurological dysfunctions (Shellhaas et al. 2017). In an investigation on children enrolled in 5 cohort studies, infants were evaluated for the pattern of their sleep at 6, 12 and 18 months of age using a parent reported questionnaire (Mindell et al. 2017). Also, social and emotional assessment was performed at 12 and 18 months of age. Their results demonstrated that more internalizing problems at 18 months of age were predictable if the child had experienced later bedtimes and less total sleep at 12 months. These internalizing problems included indices of depression/withdrawal, general anxiety, separation distress and inhibition (Mindell et al. 2017). Another large cohort study revealed that symptoms of persistent or transient sleep-disordered breathing (snoring, mouth breathing, and sleep apnea) in early life, as reported by the parents, were associated with behavioral disturbances by the ages of 4 and 7 years (Bonuck et al. 2012). In another study, researchers found that the parental report of sleep-disordered breathing or behavioral sleep problems through the first 5 years of the life increased the odds of having a special educational need when the child reaches 8 years of age (Bonuck, Rao, and Xu 2012).The other investigation revealed that inefficient sleep at 9 years of age led to the reduction of general IQ and working memory when the child became 11 years old. Also, persistent inadequate sleep during early childhood was shown to be related with reduced cognitive performance at school age (Philbrook et al. 2017). Hence, disturbed sleep patterns during early life, later bedtimes, and decreased total sleep duration not only are associated with cognitive, social and emotion problems in the child, but also are predictive of such symptoms in future.

CONCLUSION

Sleep disorders are known to affect all systems in the body (El Shakankiry 2011). In the present chapter, we mainly focused on the effects of sleep and its disturbances on the child's brain. Sleep is regulated through the interaction between several complex mechanisms. The formation and development of these mechanisms and involved neural networks in the newborn requires time and they would undergo important changes as the child grows up (Kurth et al. 2015). Multiple internal and external factors throughout the life could affect sleep regulating mechanisms; however, these mechanisms are substantially more vulnerable during first years of life (Logan et al. 2018). Hence, we could expect that sleep disorders during childhood lead to significant problems that may be persistent in adolescence and even adulthood (Meltzer 2017). Yet, far remains to be elucidated regarding the importance of sleep and subsequent disturbances associated with sleep disorders, especially in childhood (Meltzer 2017). IQ, learning, cognitive flexibility, abstract thinking, reasoning, memory, social and emotional behaviors, mental health, and school performance are some of the well-known issues proven to be linked with sleep during childhood (Philbrook et al. 2017, Telzer et al. 2015). The important role of normal sleep in childhood neurodevelopment highlights the need for effective screening of sleep disorders among children and adolescents and the critical role that early intervention and treatment could play.

REFERENCES

Angriman, M., B. Caravale, L. Novelli, R. Ferri, and O. Bruni. 2015. "Sleep in children with neurodevelopmental disabilities." *Neuropediatrics* 46 (3):199-210. doi: 10.1055/s-0035-1550151.

Barone, I., H. Hawks-Mayer, and J. O. Lipton. 2019. "Mechanisms of sleep and circadian ontogeny through the lens of neurodevelopmental disorders." *Neurobiol Learn Mem* 160:160-172. doi: 10.1016/j.nlm.2019.01.011.

Bodizs, R., F. Gombos, P. P. Ujma, and I. Kovacs. 2014. "Sleep spindling and fluid intelligence across adolescent development: sex matters." *Front Hum Neurosci* 8:952. doi: 10.3389/fnhum.2014.00952.

Bódizs, Róbert, Ferenc Gombos, Péter P. Ujma, and Ilona Kovács. 2014. *"Sleep spindling and fluid intelligence across adolescent development: sex matters."* 8 (952). doi: 10.3389/fnhum.2014.00952.

Bonuck, K., K. Freeman, R. D. Chervin, and L. Xu. 2012. "Sleep-disordered breathing in a population-based cohort: behavioral outcomes at 4 and 7 years." *Pediatrics* 129 (4):e857-65. doi: 10.1542/peds.2011-1402.

Bonuck, K., T. Rao, and L. Xu. 2012. "Pediatric sleep disorders and special educational need at 8 years: a population-based cohort study." *Pediatrics* 130 (4):634-42. doi: 10.1542/peds.2012-0392.

Brockmann, P. E., O. Bruni, L. Kheirandish-Gozal, and D. Gozal. 2019. "Reduced sleep spindle activity in children with primary snoring." *Sleep Med* 65:142-146. doi: 10.1016/j.sleep.2019.10.001.

Chu, C. J., J. Leahy, J. Pathmanathan, M. A. Kramer, and S. S. Cash. 2014. "The maturation of cortical sleep rhythms and networks over early development." *Clin Neurophysiol* 125 (7):1360-70. doi: 10.1016/j.clinph.2013.11.028.

D'Souza, D., H. D'Souza, K. Horvath, K. Plunkett, and A. Karmiloff-Smith. 2019. "Sleep is atypical across neurodevelopmental disorders in infants and toddlers: A cross-syndrome study." *Res Dev Disabil* 97:103549. doi: 10.1016/j.ridd.2019.103549.

Dahl, R. E., and D. S. Lewin. 2002. "Pathways to adolescent health sleep regulation and behavior." *J Adolesc Health* 31 (6 Suppl):175-84. doi: 10.1016/s1054-139x(02)00506-2.

Eban-Rothschild, A., L. Appelbaum, and L. de Lecea. 2018. "Neuronal Mechanisms for Sleep/Wake Regulation and Modulatory Drive." *Neuropsychopharmacology* 43 (5):937-952. doi: 10.1038/npp.2017.294.

El Shakankiry, Hanan M. 2011. "Sleep physiology and sleep disorders in childhood." *Nature and science of sleep* 3:101-114. doi: 10.2147/NSS.S22839.

Fischer, S., I. Wilhelm, and J. Born. 2007. "Developmental differences in sleep's role for implicit off-line learning: comparing children with adults." *J Cogn Neurosci* 19 (2):214-27. doi: 10.1162/jocn.2007.19.2.214.

Frank, Marcos G., Naoum P. Issa, and Michael P. Stryker. 2001. "Sleep Enhances Plasticity in the Developing Visual Cortex." *Neuron* 30 (1):275-287. doi: https://doi.org/10.1016/S0896-6273(01)00279-3.

Gomez, R. L., and J. O. Edgin. 2015. "Sleep as a window into early neural development: Shifts in sleep-dependent learning effects across early childhood." *Child Dev Perspect* 9 (3):183-189. doi: 10.1111/cdep.12130.

Institute of Medicine Committee on Sleep, Medicine, and Research. 2006. "The National Academies Collection: Reports funded by National Institutes of Health." In *Sleep Disorders and Sleep Deprivation: An Unmet Public Health Problem*, edited by H. R. Colten and B. M. Altevogt. Washington (DC): National Academies Press (US). National Academy of Sciences.

Jan, J. E., R. J. Reiter, M. C. Bax, U. Ribary, R. D. Freeman, and M. B. Wasdell. 2010. "Long-term sleep disturbances in children: a cause of neuronal loss." *Eur J Paediatr Neurol* 14 (5):380-90. doi: 10.1016/j.ejpn.2010.05.001.

Kayser, M. S., Z. Yue, and A. Sehgal. 2014. "A critical period of sleep for development of courtship circuitry and behavior in Drosophila." *Science* 344 (6181):269-74. doi: 10.1126/science.1250553.

Kocevska, Desana, Ryan L. Muetzel, Annemarie I. Luik, Maartje P. C. M. Luijk, Vincent W. Jaddoe, Frank C. Verhulst, Tonya White, and Henning Tiemeier. 2016. "The Developmental Course of Sleep Disturbances Across Childhood Relates to Brain Morphology at Age 7: The Generation R Study." *Sleep* 40 (1). doi: 10.1093/sleep/zsw022.

Kurth, S., P. Achermann, T. Rusterholz, and M. K. Lebourgeois. 2013. "Development of Brain EEG Connectivity across Early Childhood: Does Sleep Play a Role?" *Brain Sci* 3 (4):1445-60. doi: 10.3390/brainsci3041445.

Kurth, S., N. Olini, R. Huber, and M. LeBourgeois. 2015. "Sleep and Early Cortical Development." *Curr Sleep Med Rep* 1 (1):64-73. doi: 10.1007/s40675-014-0002-8.

LeBourgeois, Monique K., Douglas C. Dean, Sean C. L. Deoni, Malcolm Kohler, and Salome Kurth. 2019. "A simple sleep EEG marker in childhood predicts brain myelin 3.5 years later." *NeuroImage* 199:342-350. doi: https://doi.org/10.1016/j.neuroimage.2019.05.072.

Li, Liwen, Jiwei Ren, Lei Shi, Xinming Jin, Chonghuai Yan, Fan Jiang, Xiaoming Shen, and Shenghui Li. 2014. "Frequent nocturnal awakening in children: prevalence, risk factors, and associations with subjective sleep perception and daytime sleepiness." *BMC Psychiatry* 14 (1):204. doi: 10.1186/1471-244X-14-204.

Logan, R. W., B. P. Hasler, E. E. Forbes, P. L. Franzen, M. M. Torregrossa, Y. H. Huang, D. J. Buysse, D. B. Clark, and C. A. McClung. 2018. "Impact of Sleep and Circadian Rhythms on Addiction Vulnerability in Adolescents." *Biol Psychiatry* 83 (12):987-996. doi: 10.1016/j.biopsych.2017.11.035.

Maski, K., and J. A. Owens. 2016. "Insomnia, parasomnias, and narcolepsy in children: clinical features, diagnosis, and management." *Lancet Neurol* 15 (11):1170-81. doi: 10.1016/s1474-4422(16)30204-6.

Medic, G., M. Wille, and M. E. Hemels. 2017. "Short- and long-term health consequences of sleep disruption." *Nat Sci Sleep* 9:151-161. doi: 10.2147/nss.s134864.

Meltzer, L. J. 2017. "Sleep and Developmental Psychopathology: Introduction to the Special Issue." *J Clin Child Adolesc Psychol* 46 (2):171-174. doi: 10.1080/15374416.2016.1220316.

Mindell, J. A., E. S. Leichman, C. DuMond, and A. Sadeh. 2017. "Sleep and Social-Emotional Development in Infants and Toddlers." *J Clin Child Adolesc Psychol* 46 (2):236-246. doi: 10.1080/15374416. 2016.1188701.

Mindell, J. A., and J. A. Owens. 2003. "Sleep problems in pediatric practice: clinical issues for the pediatric nurse practitioner." *J Pediatr Health Care* 17 (6):324-31. doi: 10.1016/s0891-5245(03)00215-3.

Paruthi, S., L. J. Brooks, C. D'Ambrosio, W. A. Hall, S. Kotagal, R. M. Lloyd, B. A. Malow, K. Maski, C. Nichols, S. F. Quan, C. L. Rosen, M. M. Troester, and M. S. Wise. 2016. "Recommended Amount of Sleep for Pediatric Populations: A Consensus Statement of the American Academy of Sleep Medicine." *J Clin Sleep Med* 12 (6):785-6. doi: 10.5664/jcsm.5866.

Philbrook, L. E., J. B. Hinnant, L. Elmore-Staton, J. A. Buckhalt, and M. El-Sheikh. 2017. "Sleep and cognitive functioning in childhood: Ethnicity, socioeconomic status, and sex as moderators." *Dev Psychol* 53 (7):1276-1285. doi: 10.1037/dev0000319.

Rusterholz, T., C. Hamann, A. Markovic, S. J. Schmidt, P. Achermann, and L. Tarokh. 2018. "Nature and Nurture: Brain Region-Specific Inheritance of Sleep Neurophysiology in Adolescence." *J Neurosci* 38 (43):9275-9285. doi: 10.1523/jneurosci.0945-18.2018.

Seugnet, L., Y. Suzuki, J. M. Donlea, L. Gottschalk, and P. J. Shaw. 2011. "Sleep deprivation during early-adult development results in long-lasting learning deficits in adult Drosophila." *Sleep* 34 (2):137-46. doi: 10.1093/sleep/34.2.137.

Shellhaas, R. A., J. W. Burns, F. Hassan, M. D. Carlson, J. D. E. Barks, and R. D. Chervin. 2017. "Neonatal Sleep-Wake Analyses Predict 18-month Neurodevelopmental Outcomes." *Sleep* 40 (11). doi: 10.1093/sleep/zsx144.

Shochat, T., M. Cohen-Zion, and O. Tzischinsky. 2014. "Functional consequences of inadequate sleep in adolescents: a systematic review." *Sleep Med Rev* 18 (1):75-87. doi: 10.1016/j.smrv.2013.03.005.

Taki, Y., H. Hashizume, B. Thyreau, Y. Sassa, H. Takeuchi, K. Wu, Y. Kotozaki, R. Nouchi, M. Asano, K. Asano, H. Fukuda, and R. Kawashima. 2012. "Sleep duration during weekdays affects hippocampal gray matter volume in healthy children." *Neuroimage* 60 (1):471-5. doi: 10.1016/j.neuroimage.2011.11.072.

Tarokh, L., J. M. Saletin, and M. A. Carskadon. 2016. "Sleep in adolescence: Physiology, cognition and mental health." *Neurosci Biobehav Rev* 70:182-188. doi: 10.1016/j.neubiorev.2016.08.008.

Tashjian, S. M., D. Goldenberg, and A. Galvan. 2017. "Neural connectivity moderates the association between sleep and impulsivity in adolescents." *Dev Cogn Neurosci* 27:35-44. doi: 10.1016/j.dcn.2017.07.006.

Telzer, E. H., D. Goldenberg, A. J. Fuligni, M. D. Lieberman, and A. Galvan. 2015. "Sleep variability in adolescence is associated with altered brain development." *Dev Cogn Neurosci* 14:16-22. doi: 10.1016/j.dcn.2015.05.007.

Weisman, O., R. Magori-Cohen, Y. Louzoun, A. I. Eidelman, and R. Feldman. 2011. "Sleep-wake transitions in premature neonates predict early development." *Pediatrics* 128 (4):706-14. doi: 10.1542/peds.2011-0047.

Wilhelm, I., S. Diekelmann, and J. Born. 2008. "Sleep in children improves memory performance on declarative but not procedural tasks." *Learn Mem* 15 (5):373-7. doi: 10.1101/lm.803708.

Wilhelm, I., S. Kurth, M. Ringli, A. L. Mouthon, A. Buchmann, A. Geiger, O. G. Jenni, and R. Huber. 2014. "Sleep slow-wave activity reveals developmental changes in experience-dependent plasticity." *J Neurosci* 34 (37):12568-75. doi: 10.1523/jneurosci.0962-14.2014.

Willumsen, J., and F. Bull. 2020. "Development of WHO Guidelines on Physical Activity, Sedentary Behavior, and Sleep for Children Less Than 5 Years of Age." *J Phys Act Health* 17 (1):96-100. doi: 10.1123/jpah.2019-0457.

Zhao, Z., X. Zhao, and S. C. Veasey. 2017. "Neural Consequences of Chronic Short Sleep: Reversible or Lasting?" *Front Neurol* 8:235. doi: 10.3389/fneur.2017.00235.

Zielinski, M. R., J. T. McKenna, and R. W. McCarley. 2016. "Functions and Mechanisms of Sleep." *AIMS Neurosci* 3 (1):67-104. doi: 10.3934/Neuroscience.2016.1.67.

In: Children and Sleep
Editor: Olivie Gadbois

ISBN: 978-1-53618-074-9
© 2020 Nova Science Publishers, Inc.

Chapter 4

EMOTIONAL AND BEHAVIORAL DISTURBANCES AND SLEEP PROBLEMS IN CHILDREN

Igor A. Kelmanson[*]

Department of Children's Diseases of the Institute for Medical Education, the V.A. Almazov National Medical Research Centre, St. Petersburg, Russia
St. Petersburg State Institute of Psychology and Social Work, St. Petersburg, Russia

ABSTRACT

Disturbed sleep is commonly reported among typically developing children, and the term 'sleep-related problems' is commonly used in research in this field and can encompass a variety of issues. In cross-sectional epidemiological studies, sleep disturbances are reported in 25–45% of school-aged children. Bedtime resistance, sleep related anxiety, sleep initiation problems, insufficient hours of sleep, night waking and

---

[*] Corresponding Author's Email: iakelmanson@hotmail.com.

daytime fatigue and tiredness are sleep problems frequently reported in school aged children. The types of reported sleep problems vary with age.

An important, although insufficiently addressed issue, is possible association between sleep problems and the signs of emotional/behavioral disturbances in children. Several studies have explored the association between sleep problems and combined anxiety/depression symptomatology. Sleep problems are not currently part of the diagnostic criteria of externalizing disorders, but have been linked to aggression, attention problems, and substance use in youth. Little is currently known about associations among sleep problems and oppositional defiant disorder, although this disorder is at the intersection of internalizing and externalizing disorders and also tends to precede depression and generalized anxiety disorder.

This paper addresses possible associations between sleep disturbances in children and emotional/behavioral problems with a new look at their co-occurrences based on a suggestion that these symptoms and signs are not the emerging manifestations of an underlying disorder but rather are a network of symptoms, dynamic complex system or dynamic constellation of symptoms (and signs) that are causally interrelated.

Keywords: behavior, emotions, network analysis, sleep disturbances

Disturbed sleep is commonly reported among typically developing children, and the term 'sleep-related problems' is commonly used in research in this field (Leahy & Gradisar, 2012) and can encompass a variety of issues. In cross-sectional epidemiological studies, sleep disturbances are reported in 25–45% of school-aged children (van Litsenburg, Waumans, van den Berg, & Gemke, 2010). Bedtime resistance, sleep related anxiety, sleep initiation problems, insufficient hours of sleep, night waking and daytime fatigue and tiredness are sleep problems frequently reported in school aged children (Lipton, Becker, & Kothare, 2008; Judith A. Owens & Mindell, 2011). The types of reported sleep problems vary with age. Bedtime resistance, sleep terrors, nightmares and night waking are more common among younger children, while difficulties falling asleep, insufficient sleep duration and excessive daytime sleepiness are sleep problems more commonly reported among older children (Jenni, Fuhrer, Iglowstein, Molinari, & Largo, 2005; van Litsenburg et al., 2010).

An important, although insufficiently addressed issue, is possible association between sleep problems and the signs of emotional/behavioral disturbances in children. Several studies have explored the association between sleep problems and combined anxiety/depression symptomatology. This latter phenotype has been found to be associated with various aspects of disturbed sleep in non-clinical samples. For example, nightmares have been associated with emotional difficulties (Schredl, Fricke-Oerkermann, Mitschke, Wiater, & Lehmkuhl, 2009), while trouble sleeping was associated with parent-reported anxiety/depression in children at age 6 years and again at age 11 (Johnson, Chilcoat, & Breslau, 2000). Depressive disorders, generalized anxiety disorder and separation anxiety disorder all list sleep problems among their core symptoms. Sleep has been examined in relation to combined anxiety-depression (A. M. Gregory & O' Connor, 2002; Johnson et al., 2000), or the broader construct, 'internalizing symptoms', which includes depression and anxiety together with somatic complaints (Touchette et al., 2012). Consequently, research on sleep problems and psychopathology in the early life course has primarily focused on internalizing disorders, with a special emphasis on depression (A. M. Gregory & O' Connor, 2002).

Sleep problems are not currently part of the diagnostic criteria of externalizing disorders, but have been linked to aggression, attention problems, and substance use in youth (Alice M Gregory & Sadeh, 2012; Sadeh, Tikotzky, & Kahn, 2014). Little is currently known about associations among sleep problems and oppositional defiant disorder, although this disorder is at the intersection of internalizing and externalizing disorders and also tends to precede depression and generalized anxiety disorder (Copeland, Shanahan, Costello, & Angold, 2009).

There are different views on possible relationships between emotional and behavioral disturbances and sleep problems in children. Although present evidence rules in favor of sleep problems to predate anxiety disorders (Leahy & Gradisar, 2012), findings are supportive of both views; the same way sleep problems in childhood predicted anxiety disorders in adulthood, internalizing problems in childhood predicted insomnia in adulthood (Touchette et al., 2012) and prior anxiety disorders were associated with an increased risk of later insomnia in adolescents (Johnson, Roth, & Breslau, 2006). Correspondingly, the same way as sleep insufficiency may lead to impaired emotional processing and poorer emotional regulation (Walker & van Der Helm, 2009) troubled rumination and feeling of anxiety may activate stress responses that can override the normal sleep wake regulation and lead to difficulties with initiation and maintenance of sleep (Richardson, 2007; Saper, Cano, & Scammell, 2005). Thus a bidirectional influence is apparent; sleep and anxiety may negatively influence each other (Alice M Gregory & Sadeh, 2012). Finally, shared genetic contributions to both sleep problems and anxiety disorders have been described (Gehrman et al., 2011), as well as shared brain structures influencing both emotional regulation and sleep (Bishop, Duncan, Brett, & Lawrence, 2004; Muzur, Pace-Schott, & Hobson, 2002; Thomas et al., 2000).

Bidirectional longitudinal associations between oppositional defiant disorder and sleep problems were identified (Shanahan, Copeland, Angold, Bondy, & Costello, 2014). The literature makes it difficult to disentangle oppositional defiant disorder from attention deficit hyperactivity disorder (Mayes et al., 2008) or other disorders (Gadow, DeVincent, & Drabick, 2008). However, it is possible that some associations between externalizing disorders and sleep disturbance are, in fact, due to co-morbidity with oppositional defiant disorder. It was shown that generalized anxiety disorder/depression and oppositional defiant disorder are often co-morbid with one another, share patterns of co-morbidity with other disorders (Copeland, Angold, Costello, & Egger, 2013), and oppositional defiant disorder is, in fact, a developmental precursor of depression and generalized anxiety disorder (Rowe, Costello, Angold, Copeland, & Maughan, 2010). One core feature of these three disorders is significant irritability, which may be driven by the child's difficulty in successfully regulating negative emotions (Stringaris, Rowe, & Maughan, 2012). Children with temperamental tendencies toward being "intense", "touchy", and "easily upset" were more likely to have sleep problems (I.A. Kelmanson, 2004; Owens-Stively et al., 1997). More work is needed to clarify whether it is indeed irritability that accounts for joint associations of this cluster of psychiatric disorders with sleep problems, what role shared biological and psychosocial underpinnings play in these associations, and also how depression/generalized anxiety versus oppositional defiant disorder uniquely contribute to sleep problems and vice versa.

A new look at the co-occurrences of the sleep problems and emotional/behavioural disturbances in children might be a suggestion that these symptoms and signs are not the emerging manifestations of an underlying disorder but rather they are network of symptoms, dynamic complex system or dynamic constellation of symptoms (and signs) that are causally interrelated (Borsboom & Cramer, 2013). Based on the network model, some psychopathological disorders are conceived as a complex dynamic system. The themes of study under the network model are current topics under great expansion. Serving as a sample are works that have analyzed depressive symptomatology, comorbidity, emotional and behavioral problems (Fonseca-Pedrero, 2018). Yet, few if any attempts were made to use a network analysis in the studies on co-occurrences of sleep problems and emotional/behavioral disturbances in children.

The network analysis of possible co-occurrences between sleep disturbances, emotional and behavioral problems in children showed the strength of relationships between the variables in consideration (Igor A Kelmanson, 2019). Some variables had quite strong connections (sleep anxiety and sleep resistance; night waking and parasomnias; attention deficit/hyperactivity and oppositional defiant problems; depressive and conduct problems; depressive and anxiety problems) (Figure 1). The signs of sleep problems and emotional/behavioral disturbances in children were clustered in a specific way. So far as the emotional/behavioral features were concerned, we could identify two distinct communities of the symptoms, both by visual inspection of the network and by more rigorous explorative factor analysis: 1) attention deficit/hyperactivity and oppositional defiant problems, and 2) anxiety, conduct and depressive problems. Attention deficit/hyperactivity and oppositional defiant behavior are collectively referred to as "externalizing" behavioral disorders. Children with attention deficit/hyperactivity often have the signs of oppositional defiant behavior (disobedience and hostility towards parents, teachers or other adults), and these conditions may coexist in up 35% of children (Green, Wong, Atkins, Taylor, & Feinleib, 1999; Lahey et al., 1994). Likewise, anxiety and depressive symptoms are commonly linked and collectively referred to as "internalizing" disorders. Some authors have recommended combining depression and generalized anxiety into one "distress disorders" category (Clark & Watson, 2006; Watson, 2005). Genetic commonalities between these two disorders have also been identified (Clark & Watson, 2006). Sleep problems in children were clustering in a following way: 1) sleep anxiety and bedtime resistance; 2) night waking, parasomnias and sleep duration; 3) sleep onset delay. A tight link between sleep anxiety and sleep resistance was reported by the authors who evaluated the subscale-to-subscale correlations within the Child Sleep Habit Questionnaire (CSHQ) in clinical and community samples, and who found the highest correlations between the bedtime resistance and sleep anxiety in both samples (Judith A Owens, Spirito, & McGuinn, 2000). Furthermore, the authors who investigated daytime signs of anxiety in relation to parent-reported components of sleep difficulties found that bedtime resistance was associated with higher child-reported anxiety scores, while child anxiety was not associated with the other seven aspects of sleep problems under consideration by CSHQ, including sleep onset delay and sleep duration (Alice M Gregory, Rijsdijk, Dahl, McGuffin, & Eley, 2006). Bedtime resistance and refusal to sleep alone are commonly reported in children with the symptoms of anxiety (Alfano, Ginsburg, & Kingery, 2007; Alfano, Pina, Zerr, & Villalta, 2010).The objective sleep disturbances in children with anxiety disorders were longer sleep onset latency and less slow-wave sleep (Forbes et al., 2008). Given the association between serotonin and both sleep and anxiety (Lesch et al., 1996), it is likely that genes involved in the serotonin pathways, as well as a host of others, are likely to play a role in any sleep-anxiety relationship, some of which may be associated with internalizing difficulties (Allebrandt et al., 2013).

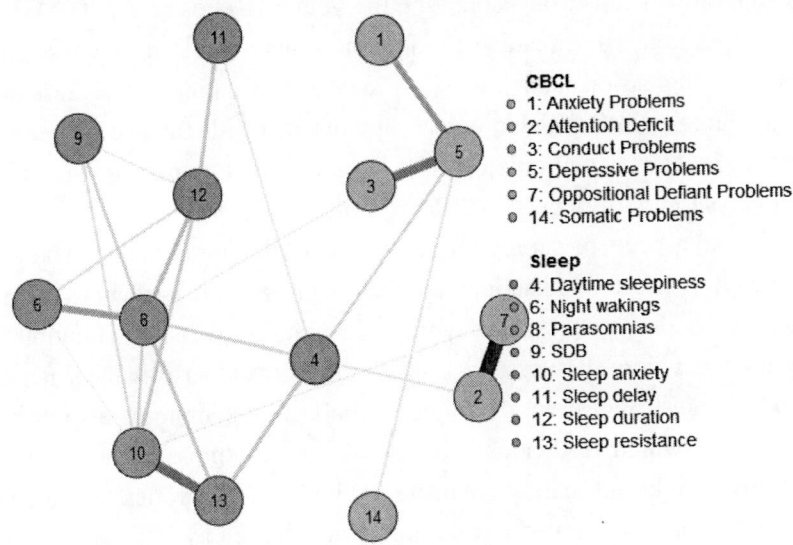

Figure 1. Network analysis of the Child Sleep Habit Questionnaire and Child Behavior Checklist (CBCL) DSM-oriented scales. Blue edges represent positive correlations, red edges – negative ones. The size and density of the edges between the nodes represent the strength of connectedness. SDS – sleep disordered breathing (Igor A Kelmanson, 2019).

Relationship between night waking, parasomnias and sleep duration problems was found (Igor A Kelmanson, 2019), and it was in accord with previous reports of the authors who supposed that the CSHQ subscales on parasomnias, sleep disordered breathing, and night waking represent other types of sleep problems, as opposed to sleep anxiety and bedtime resistance (Judith A Owens et al., 2000).

Daytime sleepiness acts as the "bridge" connecting the sleep problems and the signs of emotional disturbances (Figure 1). Excessive daytime sleepiness is commonly assumed to be the result of disturbed or inadequate sleep (Roehrs, Carskadon, Dement, & Roth, 2000). However, the literature reports a wide variety of symptoms in addition to sleep disturbance that are associated with excessive daytime sleepiness, indicating that the mechanism of excessive daytime sleepiness is a multifactorial one. In particular, excessive daytime sleepiness has been reported to be more common in patients with symptoms of depression (Chellappa & Araújo, 2006), and this association was the strongest among the young (Bixler et al., 2005). It has been suggested that circadian rhythms may play a role in the association between depression and excessive daytime sleepiness. Depression is strongly intertwined with biological rhythms on a wide range of dimensions, which includes neurobiological systems that underlie both the pathophysiology of depression, such as the serotonergic system, as well as the clinical aspects of depression. Disorders of the human circadian system can result in circadian misalignment, leading to sleep disturbances (namely, insomnia and/or excessive daytime sleepiness), reduced attention and impaired daytime alertness, lack of energy, lower performance, negative mood and gastrointestinal disorders, and all these symptoms also occur in depression, which further extends the idea that depression and circadian rhythms may be intimately connected (Chellappa, Schröder, & Cajochen, 2009). Depressive problems scale, in its turn, served as a "bridge" to some other emotional/behavioral disturbances, including anxiety, conduct and somatic problems.

Daytime sleepiness was also a "bridge" from the sleep problems to the attention deficit/hyperactivity score. Sleep problems have been associated with externalizing behavior problems such as hyperactivity and impulsivity both in cross-sectional (Aronen, Paavonen, Fjällberg, Soininen, & Törrönen, 2000; Smedje, Broman, & Hetta, 2001) and longitudinal studies (A. M. Gregory & O' Connor, 2002). Children and adolescents display increased inattentive behavior after sleep restriction (Fallone, Acebo, Seifer, & Carskadon, 2005). Children with attention deficit/hyperactivity are reported to have significantly higher bedtime resistance, more sleep onset difficulties, night waking, difficulties with morning awakenings, and display more daytime sleepiness compared to controls (Cortese, Faraone, Konofal, & Lecendreux, 2009). Studies using objective measures confirmed increased daytime sleepiness in children with attention deficit/hyperactivity (Gruber & Sadeh, 2004). Sleep insufficiency may exacerbate attention deficits and/or executive function dysfunction (Mullane, Corkum, Klein, McLaughlin, & Lawrence, 2011), and externalizing symptoms (Choi, Yoon, Kim, Chung, & Yoo, 2010). Sleep restriction has been associated with impaired performance on tests measuring sustained attention (Sadeh, Gruber, & Raviv, 2003), executive function (Randazzo, Muehlbach, Schweitzer, & Waishl, 1998), and subjectively reported sleep problems has been associated with externalizing behavior in typically developing children (Aronen et al., 2000).

The parasomnias score had strong connections with several sleep problems scores, including night waking, sleep duration, sleep resistance, sleep disordered breathing, and daytime sleepiness (Figure 1). Parasomnias are common phenomena in children; sleepwalking was reported to have occurred in 13.8%, somnoloquy (sleeptalking) in 55.5%, and bruxism (teeth grinding) in 28.1% in children aged 3–13 years (Laberge, Tremblay, Vitaro, & Montplaisir, 2000). Nightmares were reported to occur often in 2.5% and sometimes in 27.1% of children aged 8–11 years (Schredl et al., 2009). Possible link between sleep disordered breathing and parasomnias in pre-adolescent school-aged children was previously reported, and parasomnias were associated with a higher prevalence of other sleep disturbances and learning problems (Goodwin et al., 2004; Mehlenbeck, Spirito, Owens, & Boergers, 2000). The linkage between sleep disordered breathing and parasomnias most likely involves the triggering of parasomnias by arousals related to respiratory events (Espa, Dauvilliers, Ondze, Billiard, & Besset, 2002). In addition, a study in pre-pubertal children showed a clear, prompt improvement in sleepwalking and sleep talking with treatment for sleep disordered breathing and periodic limb movements, and it was suggested that both sleep disordered breathing and periodic limb movements induced parasomnias by producing brief arousals from sleep (Guilleminault, Palombini, Pelayo, & Chervin, 2003). Arousals and parasomnias lead to sleep fragmentation known as one of the leading causes of daytime sleepiness in school-aged children (Heussler, 2005).

CONCLUSION

Daytime sleepiness should be regarded as a prioritizing clinical sign in order to identify children at risk of sleep problems and associated emotional disturbances. Signs of parasomnias and depressive problems should be regarded cautiously as possible indicators of co-occurring sleep and emotional disturbances.

REFERENCES

Alfano, C. A., Ginsburg, G. S., & Kingery, J. N. (2007). Sleep-related problems among children and adolescents with anxiety disorders. *Journal of the American Academy of Child & Adolescent Psychiatry, 46*(2), 224-232.

Alfano, C. A., Pina, A. A., Zerr, A. A., & Villalta, I. K. (2010). Pre-sleep arousal and sleep problems of anxiety-disordered youth. *Child Psychiatry & Human Development, 41*(2), 156-167.

Allebrandt, K. V., Amin, N., Muller-Myhsok, B., Esko, T., Teder-Laving, M., Azevedo, R. V., ... Roenneberg, T. (2013). A K(ATP) channel gene effect on sleep duration: from genome-wide association studies to function in Drosophila. *Mol Psychiatry, 18*(1), 122-132. doi: 10.1038/mp.2011.142.

Aronen, E. T., Paavonen, E. J., Fjällberg, M., Soininen, M., & Törrönen, J. (2000). Sleep and psychiatric symptoms in school-age children. *Journal of the American Academy of Child & Adolescent Psychiatry, 39*(4), 502-508.

Bishop, S., Duncan, J., Brett, M., & Lawrence, A. D. (2004). Prefrontal cortical function and anxiety: controlling attention to threat-related stimuli. *Nature neuroscience, 7*(2), 184-188.

Bixler, E. O., Vgontzas, A. N., Lin, H. M., Calhoun, S. L., Vela-Bueno, A., & Kales, A. (2005). Excessive Daytime Sleepiness in a General Population Sample: The Role of Sleep Apnea, Age, Obesity, Diabetes, and Depression. *The Journal of Clinical Endocrinology & Metabolism, 90*(8), 4510-4515. doi: 10.1210/jc.2005-0035.

Borsboom, D., & Cramer, A. O. (2013). Network analysis: an integrative approach to the structure of psychopathology. *Annual review of clinical psychology, 9*, 91-121.

Chellappa, S. L., & Araújo, J. F. (2006). Excessive daytime sleepiness in patients with depressive disorder. *Revista Brasileira de Psiquiatria, 28*(2), 126-129.

Chellappa, S. L., Schröder, C., & Cajochen, C. (2009). Chronobiology, excessive daytime sleepiness and depression: is there a link? *Sleep Med, 10*(5), 505-514.

Choi, J., Yoon, I.-Y., Kim, H.-W., Chung, S., & Yoo, H. J. (2010). Differences between objective and subjective sleep measures in children with attention deficit hyperactivity disorder. *Journal of Clinical Sleep Medicine, 6*(06), 589-595.

Clark, L. A., & Watson, D. (2006). Distress and fear disorders: an alternative empirically based taxonomy of the 'mood'and'anxiety'disorders. *The British Journal of Psychiatry, 189*(6), 481-483.

Copeland, W. E., Angold, A., Costello, E. J., & Egger, H. (2013). Prevalence, comorbidity, and correlates of DSM-5 proposed disruptive mood dysregulation disorder. *American Journal of Psychiatry, 170*(2), 173-179.

Copeland, W. E., Shanahan, L., Costello, E. J., & Angold, A. (2009). Childhood and adolescent psychiatric disorders as predictors of young adult disorders. *Archives of general psychiatry, 66*(7), 764-772.

Cortese, S., Faraone, S. V., Konofal, E., & Lecendreux, M. (2009). Sleep in children with attention-deficit/hyperactivity disorder: meta-analysis of subjective and objective studies. *J Am Acad Child Adolesc Psychiatry, 48*(9), 894-908. doi: 10.1097/CHI.0b013e3181ac09c9.

Espa, F., Dauvilliers, Y., Ondze, B., Billiard, M., & Besset, A. (2002). Arousal reactions in sleepwalking and night terrors in adults: the role of respiratory events. *Sleep, 25*(8), 32-36.

Fallone, G., Acebo, C., Seifer, R., & Carskadon, M. A. (2005). Experimental restriction of sleep opportunity in children: effects on teacher ratings. *Sleep, 28*(12), 1561-1567.

Fonseca-Pedrero, E. (2018). Network analysis in psychology. *Psychologist Papers, 39*(1), 1-12.

Forbes, E. E., Bertocci, M. A., Gregory, A. M., Ryan, N. D., Axelson, D. A., Birmaher, B., & Dahl, R. E. (2008). Objective sleep in pediatric anxiety disorders and major depressive disorder. *Journal of the American Academy of Child & Adolescent Psychiatry, 47*(2), 148-155.

Gadow, K. D., DeVincent, C. J., & Drabick, D. A. (2008). Oppositional defiant disorder as a clinical phenotype in children with autism spectrum disorder. *Journal of Autism and Developmental Disorders, 38*(7), 1302-1310.

Gehrman, P. R., Meltzer, L. J., Moore, M., Pack, A. I., Perlis, M. L., Eaves, L. J., & Silberg, J. L. (2011). Heritability of insomnia symptoms in youth and their relationship to depression and anxiety. *Sleep, 34*(12), 1641-1646.

Goodwin, J. L., Kaemingk, K. L., Fregosi, R. F., Rosen, G. M., Morgan, W. J., Smith, T., & Quan, S. F. (2004). Parasomnias and sleep disordered breathing in Caucasian and Hispanic children–the Tucson children's assessment of sleep apnea study. *BMC medicine, 2*(1), 1-9.

Green, M., Wong, M., Atkins, D., Taylor, J., & Feinleib, M. (1999). *Diagnosis of attention-deficit/hyperactivity disorder*. Rockville, MD: Agency for Health Care Policy and Research: Technical Resources International, Inc. under Contract No. 290-94-2024.

Gregory, A. M., & O' Connor, T. G. (2002). Sleep problems in childhood: a longitudinal study of developmental change and association with behavioral problems. *J Am Acad Child Adolesc Psychiatry, 41*(8), 964-971. doi: 10.1097/00004583-200208000-00015.

Gregory, A. M., Rijsdijk, F. V., Dahl, R. E., McGuffin, P., & Eley, T. C. (2006). Associations between sleep problems, anxiety, and depression in twins at 8 years of age. *Pediatrics, 118*(3), 1124-1132.

Gregory, A. M., & Sadeh, A. (2012). Sleep, emotional and behavioral difficulties in children and adolescents. *Sleep medicine reviews, 16*(2), 129-136.

Gruber, R., & Sadeh, A. (2004). Sleep and neurobehavioral functioning in boys with attention-deficit/hyperactivity disorder and no reported breathing problems. *Sleep, 27*(2), 267-273.

Guilleminault, C., Palombini, L., Pelayo, R., & Chervin, R. D. (2003). Sleepwalking and sleep terrors in prepubertal children: what triggers them? *Pediatrics, 111*(1), e17-e25.

Heussler, H. S. (2005). Common causes of sleep disruption and daytime sleepiness: childhood sleep disorders II. *Med J Aust, 182*(9), 484-489.

Jenni, O. G., Fuhrer, H. Z., Iglowstein, I., Molinari, L., & Largo, R. H. (2005). A longitudinal study of bed sharing and sleep problems among Swiss children in the first 10 years of life. *Pediatrics, 115*(Supplement 1), 233-240.

Johnson, E. O., Chilcoat, H. D., & Breslau, N. (2000). Trouble sleeping and anxiety/depression in childhood. *Psychiatry research, 94*(2), 93-102.

Johnson, E. O., Roth, T., & Breslau, N. (2006). The association of insomnia with anxiety disorders and depression: exploration of the direction of risk. *Journal of psychiatric research, 40*(8), 700-708.

Kelmanson, I. A. (2004). Temperament and sleep characteristics in two-month-old infants. *Sleep and Hypnosis, 6*(2), 78-84.

Kelmanson, I. A. (2019). Sleep disturbances and their co-occurrence with emotional and behavioural problems in elementary school children. *Somnologie, 23*(4), 281-290.

Laberge, L., Tremblay, R. E., Vitaro, F., & Montplaisir, J. (2000). Development of parasomnias from childhood to early adolescence. *Pediatrics, 106*(1), 67-74.

Lahey, B. B., Applegate, B., Barkley, R. A., Garfinkel, B., McBurnett, K., Kerdyk, L., ... et al. (1994). DSM-IV field trials for oppositional defiant disorder and conduct disorder in children and adolescents. *Am J Psychiatry, 151*(8), 1163-1171.doi: 10.1176/ajp.151.8.1163.

Leahy, E., & Gradisar, M. (2012). Dismantling the bidirectional relationship between paediatric sleep and anxiety. *Clinical Psychologist, 16*(1), 44-56.

Lesch, K.-P., Bengel, D., Heils, A., Sabol, S. Z., Greenberg, B. D., Petri, S., ... Murphy, D. L. (1996). Association of anxiety-related traits with a polymorphism in the serotonin transporter gene regulatory region. *Science, 274*(5292), 1527-1531.

Lipton, J., Becker, R. E., & Kothare, S. V. (2008). Insomnia of childhood. *Current opinion in pediatrics, 20*(6), 641-649.

Mayes, S. D., Calhoun, S. L., Bixler, E. O., Vgontzas, A. N., Mahr, F., Hillwig-Garcia, J., ... Parvin, M. (2008). ADHD subtypes and comorbid anxiety, depression, and oppositional-defiant disorder: differences in sleep problems. *Journal of pediatric psychology, 34*(3), 328-337.

Mehlenbeck, R., Spirito, A., Owens, J., & Boergers, J. (2000). The clinical presentation of childhood partial arousal parasomnias. *Sleep Med, 1*(4), 307-312.

Mullane, J. C., Corkum, P. V., Klein, R. M., McLaughlin, E. N., & Lawrence, M. A. (2011). Alerting, orienting, and executive attention in children with ADHD. *Journal of attention disorders, 15*(4), 310-320.

Muzur, A., Pace-Schott, E. F., & Hobson, J. A. (2002). The prefrontal cortex in sleep. *Trends in cognitive sciences, 6*(11), 475-481.

Owens-Stively, J., Frank, N., Smith, A., Hagino, O., Spirito, A., Arrigan, M., & Alario, A. J. (1997). Child temperament, parenting discipline style, and daytime behavior in childhood sleep disorders. *Journal of Developmental and Behavioral Pediatrics, 18*(5), 314-321.

Owens, J. A., & Mindell, J. A. (2011). Pediatric Insomnia. *Pediatric Clinics, 58*(3), 555-569. doi: 10.1016/j.pcl.2011.03.011.

Owens, J. A., Spirito, A., & McGuinn, M. (2000). The Children's Sleep Habits Questionnaire (CSHQ): psychometric properties of a survey instrument for school-aged children. *Sleep - New York, 23*(8), 1043-1052.

Randazzo, A. C., Muehlbach, M. J., Schweitzer, P. K., & Waishl, J. K. (1998). Cognitive function following acute sleep restriction in children ages 10–14. *Sleep, 21*(8), 861-868.

Richardson, G. S. (2007). Human physiological models of insomnia. *Sleep Med, 8 Suppl 4*, S9-14. doi: 10.1016/s1389-9457(08)70003-0.

Roehrs, T., Carskadon, M., Dement, W., & Roth, T. (2000). Daytime sleepiness and alertness. In M. Kryger, T. Roth & W. Dement (Eds.), *Principles and practice of sleep medicine* (3rd ed., pp. 43-52). Philadelphia: WB Saunders Co.

Rowe, R., Costello, E. J., Angold, A., Copeland, W. E., & Maughan, B. (2010). Developmental pathways in oppositional defiant disorder and conduct disorder. *Journal of abnormal psychology, 119*(4), 726-738.

Sadeh, A., Gruber, R., & Raviv, A. (2003). The effects of sleep restriction and extension on school- age children: What a difference an hour makes. *Child development, 74*(2), 444-455.

Sadeh, A., Tikotzky, L., & Kahn, M. (2014). Sleep in infancy and childhood: implications for emotional and behavioral difficulties in adolescence and beyond. *Current opinion in psychiatry, 27*(6), 453-459.

Saper, C. B., Cano, G., & Scammell, T. E. (2005). Homeostatic, circadian, and emotional regulation of sleep. *Journal of Comparative Neurology, 493*(1), 92-98.

Schredl, M., Fricke-Oerkermann, L., Mitschke, A., Wiater, A., & Lehmkuhl, G. (2009). Longitudinal study of nightmares in children: stability and effect of emotional symptoms. *Child psychiatry and human development, 40*(3), 439-449.

Shanahan, L., Copeland, W. E., Angold, A., Bondy, C. L., & Costello, E. J. (2014). Sleep problems predict and are predicted by generalized anxiety/depression and oppositional defiant disorder. *Journal of the American Academy of Child & Adolescent Psychiatry, 53*(5), 550-558.

Smedje, H., Broman, J.-E., & Hetta, J. (2001). Associations between disturbed sleep and behavioural difficulties in 635 children aged six to eight years: a study based on parents' perceptions. *European child & adolescent psychiatry, 10*(1), 1-9.

Stringaris, A., Rowe, R., & Maughan, B. (2012). Mood dysregulation across developmental psychopathology—general concepts and disorder specific expressions. *Journal of Child Psychology and Psychiatry, 53*(11), 1095-1097.

Thomas, M., Sing, H., Belenky, G., Holcomb, H., Mayberg, H., Dannals, R., . . . Rowland, L. (2000). Neural basis of alertness and cognitive performance impairments during sleepiness. I. Effects of 24 h of sleep deprivation on waking human regional brain activity. *Journal of sleep research, 9*(4), 335-352.

Touchette, E., Chollet, A., Galéra, C., Fombonne, E., Falissard, B., Boivin, M., & Melchior, M. (2012). Prior sleep problems predict internalising problems later in life. *Journal of affective disorders, 143*(1-3), 166-171.

van Litsenburg, R. R. L., Waumans, R. C., van den Berg, G., & Gemke, R. J. (2010). Sleep habits and sleep disturbances in Dutch children: a population-based study. *European journal of pediatrics, 169*(8), 1009-1015.

Walker, M. P., & van Der Helm, E. (2009). Overnight therapy? The role of sleep in emotional brain processing. *Psychological bulletin, 135*(5), 731-748.

Watson, D. (2005). Rethinking the mood and anxiety disorders: a quantitative hierarchical model for DSM-V. *Journal of abnormal psychology, 114*(4), 522-536.

In: Children and Sleep
Editor: Olivie Gadbois

ISBN: 978-1-53618-074-9
© 2020 Nova Science Publishers, Inc.

Chapter 5

FROM MOUTH BREATHING TO PEDIATRIC OBSTRUCTIVE SLEEP APNEA: CONSEQUENCES, DIAGNOSIS AND TREATMENT OPTIONS

Maria Christina Thomé Pacheco[1,*]*,*
Fabiana Vasconcelos Campos[2]
and Maria Teresa Martins de Araújo[2]

[1]Department of Dental Clinic, Federal University of Espírito Santo,
Vitória – ES, Brazil
[2]Department of Physiological Sciences,
Federal University of Espírito Santo. Vitória – ES, Brazil

ABSTRACT

Pediatric obstructive sleep apnea (OSA) is – much like in the adult form of the disease – caused by the abnormal blockage of the upper airway during sleep. As a rather pliant conduit, the upper airway is naturally

---
[*] Corresponding Author's Email: mchristp@gmail.com.

subject to collapsing, becoming even more so during sleep and when extrinsic factors, such as craniofacial alterations and breathing disorders, are in place.

The shaping of the palate and upper airway structures begins with the sucking and swallowing that take place *in utero*. At birth and during early childhood, the coordination between sucking, swallowing, chewing and nasal breathing plays a significant role in the development of the human face, affecting the expansion of craniofacial structures and the shape taken by the upper airway.

Breathing disorders involving obstruction of the upper airway are often the reason why children breathe through their mouths. The persistence of mouth breathing throughout the development compromises facial bones and the positioning of teeth, affecting the stomatognathic system and even the body's posture. Thus, if a child does not breathe properly, she cannot swallow, chew or talk so.

The younger the child at the onset of such sleep-related breathing disorders, the more severe the outcome later in life. Therefore, an early diagnosis of pediatric OSA through the identification of potential risk factors could, at the very least, decrease the impact this particular disorder has over the lives of afflicted subjects. It is, however, rather more complicated to diagnose OSA in children than in the adult population, save in cases when the symptoms are particularly severe. An integrated, multidisciplinary approach is, therefore, necessary not only to diagnose but also to treat the pediatric form of this disease.

This chapter addresses the details on how the replacement of nasal breathing by mouth breathing in childhood affects the development of facial structures and the upper airway, compromising the dental arches and making children more vulnerable to OSA.

We will discuss the consequences of persistent mouth breathing and upper airway obstructions, as well as of deleterious oral habits and the very body posture adopted by the child. We shall then focus on the main causes underlying sleep-disordered breathing, along with a detailed review on clinical procedures and complementary exams that, combined with the indispensable polysomnography with capnography, assist in the difficult diagnosis of OSA in children. Finally, we will conduct a thorough discussion on treatment options available for such patients.

With this chapter, we endeavor to highlight the importance of identifying the causes behind the development of mouth breathing and OSA in children, for, if left untreated, such breathing disorders can progress to more severe conditions in adulthood.

INTRODUCTION

The shaping of the palate and upper airway (UA) begins during intrauterine life, as the fetus starts swallowing and sucking. At birth and during early childhood, the coordination between nasal breathing, sucking, swallowing and chewing are crucial for the development of the human face, directing the expansion of craniofacial structures and the shape taken by the UA [1].

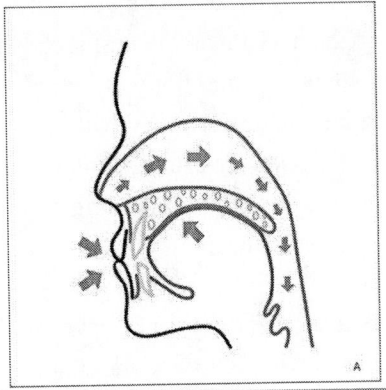

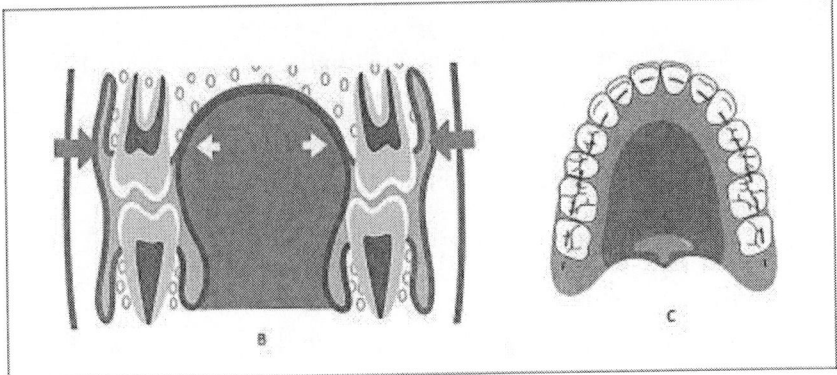

Figure 1. A-C. Regular nasal breathing. (A) Lips are sealed and the tongue touches the palate. (B) Internal and external muscle forces are balanced in the mouth. (C) Shape of the maxilla and dental arch are in equilibrium.

Nasal breathing is the main function underlying the three-dimensional development of the sinuses and nasal fossae, whose base forms the roof of the oral cavity. The balance between the air entering the nose, the sealing of the lips and the position of the tongue dorsum against the hard palate stimulates the anterior and transverse growth of maxillary bones, increasing the volume of nasal and oral cavities.

The muscles of the face also have great influence on bone and dental tissues, as well as on their supporting structures. Thus, when one breathes through the nose, the balance between internal and external forces applied by the muscles helps with the positioning of the teeth (Figure 1). Moreover, during nose-breathing, the resting posture assumed by the tongue on the roof of the oral cavity acts by naturally expanding the hard palate, assisting in the normal development of the maxilla and dental arch [1].

The relationship between maxillary bones, tongue and posterior pharyngeal wall determine the uniformity of the UA diameter. The pharynx controls the respiratory function by establishing a certain free diameter for the airflow directed to the lungs. Maintaining this diameter requires an adequate tone of the intrinsic musculature of the pharynx itself, as well as from its supporting muscles. Elastic tensile forces of the tracheobronchial system, which is connected to the tongue via larynx and hyoid bone, promote the downward displacement of the larynx and diaphragm during inspiration [1].

The anatomical and functional integrity of the airway promoted by nasal breathing is essential for proper craniofacial growth and development. Mechanical or functional obstructions of the airflow in the airway force the child to interrupt nasal breathing, breathing through the mouth in order to maintain her vital functions.

The persistence of mouth breathing during the child's growth phase compromises the entire stomatognathic system, being closely related to deleterious oral habits, UA obstruction, changes in the facial skeleton, positioning of teeth and the body's posture. Over time, there is a progressive worsening of the UA in its altered shape, along with the worsening of sleep-related obstructive breathing disorders [2].

Sleep-disordered breathing in children is characterized by a continuum that goes from snoring to respiratory effort-related arousal (RERA), culminating in obstructive sleep apnea (OSA), which is the repetitive, total or partial obstruction of the UA. The UA is no more than a rather flexible tube, being thus naturally prone to collapsing. The probability of that happening may be increased by both intrinsic and extrinsic factors. Amid the extrinsic ones, fat deposits (more present in adults), hypertrophy of the tonsils and craniofacial anatomical alterations are known to affect UA conformation, with the last two being found more often in children.

UA obstructions in childhood, particularly the hypertrophy of the tonsils, are behind most of the breathing disorders that force a child to breathe through the mouth, increasing the risk of abnormal development of bone structures that support the UA. Thus, breathing predominantly through the mouth may lead to craniofacial growth alterations, increasing the risk of disordered breathing during sleep and UA collapse. This outcome has greater impact during early childhood, for much of the development of the human face occurs between birth and the early years of life [2].

Therefore, the organism of a child who breathes predominantly through the mouth may suffer a number of consequences: if a child does not breathe properly, she cannot chew, swallow or speak so.

MOUTH BREATHING AND DELETERIOUS HABITS

Historically, mouth breathing has been signaled as an important etiological factor for changes in facial growth, with the first experiments designed to test this relationship being conducted by [3]. These authors blocked the nostrils of young Rhesus monkeys with silicone plugs and evaluated the resulting adaptive skeletal and dental modifications. They observed several types of malocclusions, depending on the adaptation imposed by muscles recruited by the animal in order to breathe through the mouth. The most relevant ones were anterior open bite, maxillary or mandibular protrusion, tongue interposition, groove formation on the tongue dorsum, shortening of the upper lip, anterior crossbite and constriction of the maxilla. However, all animals displayed an increase in the vertical growth of the face, characterized by downward rotation of the mandible. That resulted in an increase of the anterior facial height and the angle between the base of the skull and the mandible, as well as in the opening of the gonial angle and in the extrusion of posterior teeth. These skeletal alterations were perpetuated even after the nasal obstruction was removed, leading to the conclusion that changes in neuromuscular recruitment patterns trigger function and posture alterations in the mandible, tongue and upper lip [3, 4].

Despite the many reports made at that time, there was still great disbelief regarding the association between airway obstruction and changes in facial growth. The different craniofacial alterations caused by the change from nasal to mouth breathing puzzled the specialists, who expected a single adaptive pattern to characterize the mouth breather.

Causes for the development of mouth breathing	
Newborns	Choanal atresia Nasal tumors (dermoid cyst, hemangioma)
Childhood	Hypertrophy of the adenoid Hypertrophy of the palatine tonsils Allergic rhinitis Nasal septum deviation
Puberty	Tumors such as juvenile nasal angiofibroma Nasal polyps Drug-induced rhinitis Nasal septum deviation

Figure 2. Causes for the development of mouth breathing.

The most frequent airway obstructions in the nasal cavity are inferior turbinate hypertrophy and septum deviation, while in the posterior part of the nasal and oral cavities the hypertrophy of the adenoid and palatine tonsils are the most frequent airway obstructions in the nasopharynx and oropharynx, respectively. There is ample evidence showing that the hypertrophy of the adenoid is the most common cause of UA obstruction in children, followed by inferior nasal turbinate hypertrophy [5]. Often, the outcome of the alterations brought about by mouth breathing will depend on the age at which the airway obstruction was acquired, its severity and duration.

The causes of airway obstruction that may lead to mouth breathing are many and can be classified according to age group (Figure 2).

In order to keep the mouth open during mouth breathing, the child opens her lips and lowers the mandible. This simple adaptive behavior is in itself capable of promoting an imbalance between internal and external oral muscles, causing facial and dental skeletal deformities, especially during the period of facial growth. While the mouth remains open, the tongue assumes a lower position toward the oral floor to allow airflow, no longer shaping the palate and nasal base. As a consequence, the palate loses the stimulus given by the tongue to grow laterally, becoming narrow or constricted, which also inhibits the growth in width of the nasal base. On the other hand, the musculature of the face continues to act on the maxillary complex. While contracted, the buccinator muscle maintains the palate narrowed, altering bone growth and the position of the teeth in the upper dental arch from a parabolic to a triangular shape (Figure 3), which leads to a constricted maxilla. If the mouth remains persistently open, a continuous eruption of the posterior teeth will take place, while the tongue – in its low, forward position – prevents the eruption of the anterior teeth, leading to the malocclusion known as anterior open bite. In addition, the low posture assumed by the tongue widens the dentoalveolar portion of the mandible, widening the mandibular dental arch as opposed to the narrow width of the maxillary arch, which may give rise to an inverted bite known as the posterior crossbite. Parted lips and altered tongue posture induce the anterior projection of the incisors. As a result, the whole face grows more vertically, becoming elongated (Figure 4). Individuals with prolonged mouth breathing present alterations such as vertical enlargement of the lower third of the face, constricted palate, anterior open bite, posterior crossbite, obtuse gonial angle, protruded upper incisors, short upper lip, everted lower lip, hypotonia of the mandibular elevator muscles, hypotonia of the tongue, changes in tongue posture at rest and in body posture [6]. The musculoskeletal consequences on mouth breathers were evaluated in studies conducted by our research group. We found a high prevalence of constricted palate (53.9%), an absence of lip sealing (35.9%) and the presence of anterior open bite (23.4%) in mouth breathers. We have also found an increase in the vertical growth of the face – long face (34.7%) – in the afflicted subjects [7, 8].

A child who breathes through the mouth may do so due to obstructive causes, i.e., when there are mechanical obstacles hindering or impeding nasal breathing. But mouth breathing can also be a habit, persisting even after the removal of mechanical, pathological or functional obstacles, not to mention that in some cases it may happen as a result of neurological dysfunctions [9].

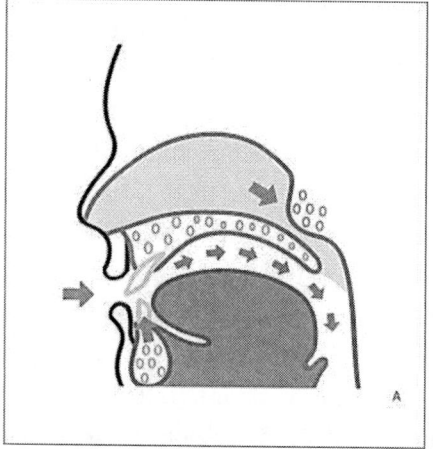

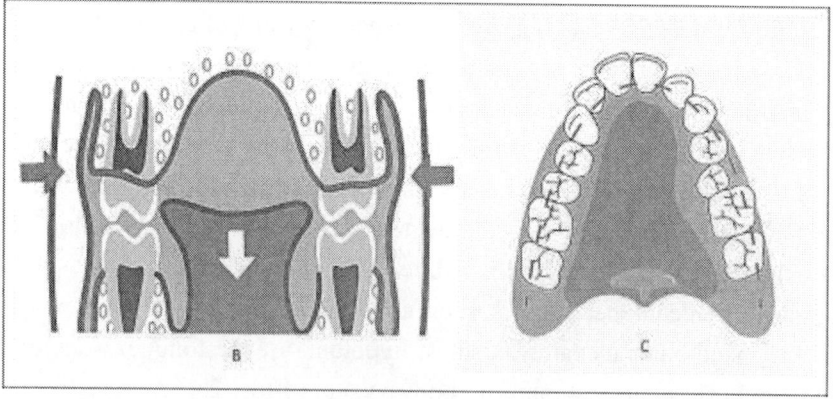

Figure 3. A-C. Mouth breathing. (A) Parted lips and tongue in a lower position to allow airflow through the mouth. (B) Imbalance between internal and external muscle forces in the mouth. (C) Skeletal alterations in the maxilla and in the shape of the dental arch.

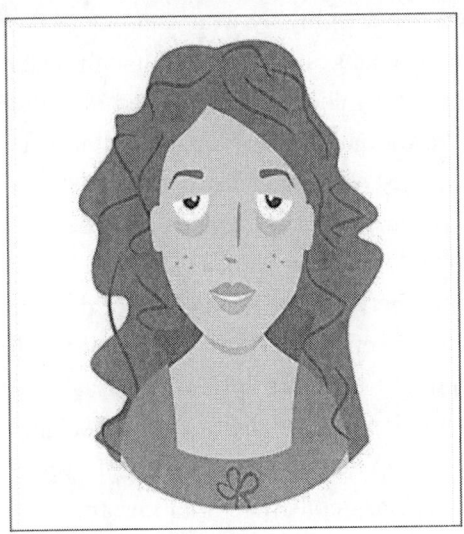

Figure 4. Typical face of a mouth breathing child - long face shape.

Generally speaking, exclusive mouth breathing is quite rare, with a mixed pattern of mouth and nasal breathing being observed most of the time [9]. The fact remains that, if the UA is at least partially obstructed, one is compelled to breathe through the mouth. After a prolonged period of mouth breathing, the person acquires the habit of breathing through the mouth, continuing to do so in the presence of the obstruction and even after its removal. Such habit is an involuntary and pleasurable action for those who practice it. However, much like every habit, once acquired it is difficult to let it go. Its persistence can be explained by the greater amount of air that enters the mouth compared to the airflow through the nose. Besides, it is actually easier to breathe so. Therefore, it is imperative to re-educate the way the individual breathes, so that he or she can switch back to nose breathing.

The most significant consequences of mouth breathing take place in childhood. Facial growth is mainly influenced by genetic factors, though environmental aspects, such as nasal breathing, do contribute to normal growth. Persistent environmental changes alter facial growth, making it amenable to various adaptations. Oral habits considered deleterious are mouth breathing and non-nutritive sucking, which include finger, pacifier and bottle sucking, tongue or lip interposition between the teeth. The persistence of these habits is highly worrying due to the facial, functional, postural and emotional changes involved. Although such habits are common until the age of three, they should be abolished in early childhood, for the child's face is still in formation, becoming fully formed only after puberty. Moreover, most acquired skeletal changes do not self-correct. Our research group found a prevalence of 37% of some type of deleterious oral habit still active in a group of children from 7 to 13 years old. In addition, a significant association was found between the persistence of deleterious habits and the presence of airway obstruction such as hypertrophic palatine tonsils, inferior turbinate hypertrophy, absence of lip sealing, nasal septum deviation and obstructive Mallampati score. A significant association was also found between the persistence of deleterious habits and the presence of craniofacial changes, such as maxillary constriction and protrusion, anterior open bite and posterior crossbite [10].

If mouth breathing is not eliminated, postural adaptations resulting from either obstructive or habitual mouth breathing will be the same, and so will the resulting facial and dental skeletal changes. And during the growth phase, not only the craniofacial development can be impaired by mouth breathing, but so could the body's posture, which may affect organs and systems [6].

In an attempt to increase the patency of the UA to ease the airflow through the mouth, one of the main postural alterations that take place is the forward head posture. This projection of the head compromises both the orofacial musculature, with changes in mandible, hyoid bone and tongue posture, as well as the sternocleidomastoid, scalene and pectoral muscles, which become shortened due to increased cervical lordosis. In addition to the forward head posture, the mouth breather protrudes the shoulders and elevates the scapulae (protruding scapulae) – an asymmetric thoracic kyphosis –, increasing lumbar lordosis and the anterior projection of the pelvis [11]. This lordotic posture associated with pelvic anteversion contributes to abdominal protrusion [11, 12, 13]. Due to the synergistic performance of the muscles and the fact that they are organized in chains (anterior and posterior), a postural alteration will result in compromised body posture as the body attempts to seek compensations [13].

The persistence of mouth breathing also leads to changes in the functioning of the temporomandibular joint (TMJ). TMJ dysfunction is one of the imbalances in muscle forces observed with persistent mouth breathing. Increased loading of the TMJ condyle and increased occipital nerve compression result in neck and shoulder muscle fatigue [14]. Nerve compression and TMJ alterations may be responsible for headaches and hyperactivity, as well as shoulder, neck, mandible and head muscle pain [15, 16]. Our research group found that mouth breathing children had a significantly higher chance of presenting masticatory and TMJ alterations, such as: mandibular deviation, limitation or pain during mandibular movements, clicking, pain in the masticatory muscles upon palpation, pain in the TMJ region, facial asymmetry and apparent muscular hypertrophy [17]. In yet another study, we evaluated the association between the presence of masticatory and TMJ alterations with the perception of mouth breathing children as to sleeping, eating and learning. We found that when mandibular deviation in opening and protruding were present, these children were more likely to report waking up with a dry mouth. Also, mouth breathers with severe overjet reported having greater learning difficulties when compared to those who did not present this occlusal alteration [18].

The postural compensation adopted by a mouth breathing child interferes with the mechanics of breathing. Malfunctioning of neck and thorax muscles results in not only anatomical but also in functional dysfunctions, with breathing becoming short and rapid and progressing to a more apical ventilatory pattern. This pattern is reinforced by the fact that the diaphragm and abdominal muscles have become hypotonic, so much so that the effectiveness of the diaphragm, which relies on the stability of the abdominal wall to support the viscera during inspiration, is impaired. This deficiency, along with the instability of the lumbar paravertebral muscles – which enable the vertebral insertion of the diaphragm –, causes a reduction of the diaphragmatic apposition zone, altering the thoracoabdominal dynamics [19, 20]. On top of that, nasal afferent nerves, which are responsible for regulating lung capacity and volume, may be inhibited, resulting in inadequate use of respiratory muscles and progressive muscle weakness [13]. Our research group has also shown that the presence of a thoracic breathing pattern and the use of accessory muscles increased in about four-fold the chance that children thus afflicted would present mouth breathing, when these parameters were compared to those of children who breathed through the nose [21].

It may seem natural to use the oral passage as an airway, but it is not. The mouth has its function in feeding and the nose in breathing. Just as it is not possible to feed through the nose, one should not be allowed to breathe through the mouth, except as a survival mechanism.

Pediatric Obstructive Sleep Apnea

The complexity of the problems that mouth breathing imposes on the individual's development has come to be better understood only in recent decades. We now known that mouth breathing during sleep – which may or may not be associated with lack of anatomical and functional integrity of the UA, with facial anatomical alterations, allergies or colds – may be a causal factor in the occurrence of obstructive sleep apnea in childhood [2]. Similarly, in adults, mouth breathing during sleep increases the resistance to airflow through the upper airway, being associated with a marked increase in the severity of obstructive sleep apnea also in this population [22, 23].

Obstructive sleep-disordered breathing may occur in children and adults, and include snoring, respiratory effort-related arousal (RERA), and obstructive sleep apnea (OSA) [24]. The so-called primary snoring is taken as a benign condition without physiological alterations or associated complications. Habitual snoring, on the other hand, happens at least 4 times a week and may be associated with other breathing problems. RERA is a sequence of breaths characterized by a progressive increase in the respiratory effort that leads to awakening in the absence of apnea or hypopnea, being currently considered a continuity of the clinical signs between habitual snoring and OSA. Pediatric OSA, on the other hand, is associated with snoring, sleep fragmentation, excessive daytime sleepiness, obstructive hypoventilation and hypercapnia, and reduced neurocognitive performance [25]. The prevalence of OSA in children ranges from 1 to 4%, being higher in boys, overweight children, those of African descent, and those with a history of atopy and prematurity [26].

Sleep apnea can be perceived by family members when the child presents habitual snoring, when she suffers respiratory arrests (apneas) and when she sleeps in a restless way. However, other symptoms may be observed, i.e., mouth breathing, intense movement during sleep, excessive sweating, enuresis, cognitive and behavioral changes, such as attention deficit and hyperactivity. These can cause learning impairment and poor school performance and, more rarely, excessive sleepiness [27]. Although some children do not display the classic snoring, they may have noisy and difficult breathing, mouth breathing, frequent episodes of upper respiratory tract infection and otitis media.

Signs and symptoms related to OSA in children	
Nocturnal	Habitual snoring (> 4 nights/week) Respiratory arrest episodes (apnea) Respiratory discomfort Restlessness Excessive sweating Cyanosis/pallor
Diurnal	Hyperactivity Difficulty in paying attention Aggressive behavior Excessive daytime sleepiness Learning problems Mouth breathing

Figure 5. Signs and symptoms related to OSA in children.

During childhood there is a higher incidence of infectious processes of the UA, as well as the overgrowth of the lymphoid tissues, leading to reduced airway diameter and consequent airflow impairment. The hypertrophy of the adenoid and palatine tonsils is considered the most important risk factor for the development of OSA in childhood [28]. Such prolonged obstruction can lead to numerous consequences according to its intensity and time of evolution, and when the child sleeps, it may increase with the relaxation of UA muscles and tongue collapse, favoring OSA [6]. In addition to adeno-tonsillar hypertrophy, craniofacial alterations, a few genetic syndromes, neurological diseases, among others, are also associated with a higher prevalence of OSA in children [29, 30]. The main signs and symptoms of pediatric OSA are shown in Figure 5.

OSA leads to consequences that impact physical, psychological (emotional) and social conditions of affected children in a negative way. Among the main comorbidities observed are pulmonary hypertension, which may progress to *cor pulmonale*, and cardiovascular alterations. The mechanisms leading to these alterations are most likely related to the interaction between intermittent hypoxia, hypercapnia, frequent arousals, and variations in intrathoracic pressures. Similar to adults, children have shown elevation of nocturnal blood pressure, changes in left ventricular geometry and function, and maintenance of sympathetic nervous system activity during wakefulness, which contributes to daytime systemic arterial hypertension. A progression of the systemic inflammatory process and an alteration in lipid metabolism have also been verified, with these events being linked to the propagation of atherogenesis and endothelial alteration processes [31].

Several reports describe the association between OSA and hyperactivity, lack of attention, aggressiveness and oppositional behavior. Strong evidence points to pediatric OSA being associated with impaired attention, behavior, emotion regulation, academic performance, and alertness. OSA also affects mood, language expression skills, visual perception and memory [32, 33]. Experimental studies on animals of different ages show that intermittent hypoxia leads to alterations in spatial memory, hyperactivity and neuronal apoptosis in the prefrontal cortex, with the age of animals showing the most affected memory corresponding to the preschool period in humans [34, 35].

Sleep fragmentation compromises the child's wakefulness, who may also have daytime sleepiness, which contributes to the inability in performing physical and learning activities. Daytime sleepiness associated with constant low functional oxygenation lead children to display behavioral alterations that also compromise the learning process, as well as the emotional development, self-esteem and socialization. Cerebral hypoxemia leads to mental tiredness, poor attention span, impaired comprehension and poor school productivity [35]. Poor school performance or learning disabilities are the result of specific difficulties involving oral language, slow reading and writing acquisition [36].

It is worthy of note that identifying the causes that may contribute to the development of mouth breathing and OSA in children is of paramount importance, for undiagnosed or untreated breathing disorders in childhood may progress to severe apnea in adulthood [37].

CLINICAL DIAGNOSIS

The diagnosis of sleep-related breathing disorders is based upon clinical and imaging criteria, brought forward by different healthcare fields, i.e., medicine, dentistry, speech and physical therapy. Clinical examination evaluates organic and functional, dentoskeletal and myofunctional features, as well as the osteomyofascial (posture) and respiratory systems.

The complementary exams most frequently employed in the diagnosis of breathing disorders are cavum and sinus radiography, nasofibroscopy, lateral cephalometric radiography (LCR), computed tomography, nuclear magnetic resonance and polysomnography.

The family history of allergic rhinitis, asthma, urticaria, anaphylaxis, food allergy and medication use should also be carefully investigated. A diagnosis is made when evidence confirming immune disorders are found through tests such as IgE titration and skin tests performed with various allergen extracts [38].

Clinical examination evaluates the nasal cavities and paranasal sinuses by rhinoscopy; the external acoustic meatus and the presence of tympanic membrane retraction by otoscopy; the oral cavity and the presence of palatine tonsil hypertrophy by oroscopy. The latter evaluates the degree of narrowing of the UA passage in the retropalatal region by the degree of palatine tonsil hypertrophy [39], which identifies the narrowing of the airway in the transverse direction (Figures 6-7). The modified Mallampati score [40], on the other hand, evaluates the distance between the uvula and the tongue dorsum with the mouth open and the tongue relaxed inside it, a position considered more natural and physiological. This parameter identifies the narrowing of the UA in the vertical direction (Figures 8-9). Brodsky degrees 3 and 4 and Mallampati score classes III and IV are considered obstructive.

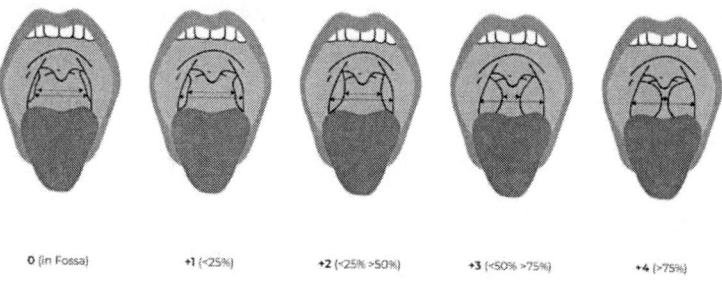

Figure 6. Brodsky classification for the palatine tonsils.

Brodsky Classification	
Degree of tonsils obstruction	Ratio of the tonsils in the oropharynx
Degree 0	Tonsils in the fossa
Degree 1	Tonsils occupy less than 25% of the oropharynx
Degree 2	Tonsils occupy from 25 to 50% of the oropharynx
Degree 3	Tonsils occupy from 51 to 75% of the oropharynx
Degree 4	Tonsils occupy more than 75% of the oropharynx

Figure 7. Brodsky classification.

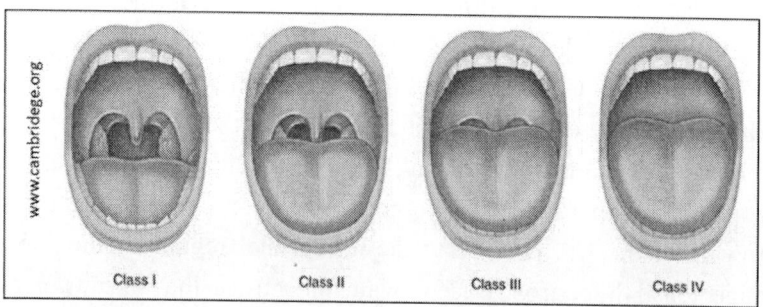

Figure 8. Modified Mallampati score; source: http://www.cambridge.org.

Modified Mallampati Classification	
Scores	Soft palate/tongue relationship
Class I	Soft palate, uvula, fauces and faucial pillars visible
Class II	Soft palate, fauces and uvula visible
Class III	Soft palate and base of the uvula visible
Class IV	Uvula not at all visible

Figure 9. Modified Mallampati classification.

Facial morphology is directly examined with the aid of a caliper or a graded ruler. This assessment considers the relationship between morphological facial height and bizygomatic width, as well as facial depth. Individuals classified as brachyfacials show greater width in relation to facial height, while in those classified as dolichofacials, height predominates over facial width. Facial symmetry, as well as facial proportions in the upper, middle and lower thirds of the face is also considered, being assessed in the frontal and profile views, with the individual's head in a natural position. There should be a proportional relationship between the facial thirds: upper (hairline to eyebrow), medium (eyebrow to subnasal point) and lower (subnasal point to the soft tissues of the chin). The symmetry between the right and left sides of the individual (frontal norm) in both width and height is also assessed. One should check for lip sealing, lip and chin tonicity and the relationship between upper and lower jaws. Good lip sealing suggests absence of vertical and sagittal skeletal discrepancies, adequate lip lengths, and lower facial height proportional to maxillary and mandible sizes, normal breathing function, and normal lip tonicity. Individuals with retrognathism may present absence of lip sealing, interposition of the lower lip between teeth, and forced lip sealing with hypertrophy of the mentalis muscle. In lateral norm, they present a convex profile and a short chin-neck line in the anteroposterior direction. Vertically they may present an acute chin-neck angle, which is indicative of a more vertical facial growth pattern [41].

Intraoral examination is performed by assessing the anteroposterior, transverse and vertical relationship between the teeth and the upper and lower jaws. In the anteroposterior relationship, a Class I occurs when maxilla and mandible are in harmony within the face; a Class II occurs when the mandible is retruded in relation to the maxilla; and a Class III when the maxilla is retruded in relation to the mandible. The same classification is applied to the dental relationship between the arches. In the transverse relationship, one evaluates whether there is jaw constriction or any inverted bite, classified as posterior crossbite. In the vertical relationship, one verifies if the anterior superior teeth cover 1/3 of the inferior teeth (overbite). Lack of overbite classifies an anterior open bite, while excess overbite classifies a deep bite [41].

Functional examination as breathing, swallowing and tongue posture during function is also performed. Our research group has put forward a set of measures for the clinical recognition of mouth breathing in children through visual assessment, by interviewing the parents and/or the child and through breathing tests, as shown in Figure 10 [8]. The recommended breathing tests are the graded mirror (Figure 11), mouth water retention, and lip sealing. The last two consist of checking if the child (without obstruction in the UA) can keep the lips sealed for up to three minutes.

Clinical identification of mouth breathing in children		
1. Visual evaluation	**2. Questions**	**3. Respiratory tests**
The dentist should investigate the presence of the following traits:	To be answered by the parents or the child herself.	At least two of the following tests should be performed, with the child in a sitting position.
With the child standing up:	Do you:	**a. Graded mirror test**
Lips remain open. Yes / No	Sleep with your mouth open? Yes / No	The child should breathe on the mirror and the second condensation halo outlined with a marking pen (figure). Low nasal flow: < 30mm; average nasal flow: 30-60mm; high nasal flow: > 60mm.
Posture alterations. Yes / No	Keep your mouth open when distracted? Yes / No	**b. Water retention test**
Dark circles under the eyes. Yes / No	Snore? Yes / No	Water should be poured in the child's mouth (approximately 15mL) and held there for 3 minutes.
Elongated face. Yes / No	Drool on your pillow? Yes / No	**c. Lip seal test**
With the child sitting down:	Present excessive daytime sleepiness? Yes / No	The child's mouth should be sealed with masking tape for 3 minutes.
Anterior open bite. Yes / No	Wake up with a headache? Yes / No	
High narrow palate. Yes / No	Get tired easily? Yes / No	
Gingivitis in maxillary incisors. Yes / No	Suffer from allergies often? Yes / No	
	Get a stuffy or runny nose often? Yes / No	
	Have difficulties at school? Yes / No	
	Have concentration problems? Yes / No	
4. Lip sealing routine to eliminate the habit of mouth breathing		
The child's mouth should be sealed with masking tape when she is distracted or has her attention focused elsewhere. The amount of time the lips remain sealed should be increased progressively each day, until the child is able to breathe only through the nose for at least 2 consecutive hours. The routine should be carried out at home on a daily basis until the child is able to return to nose breathing.		

Figure 10. Clinical identification of mouth breathing in children.

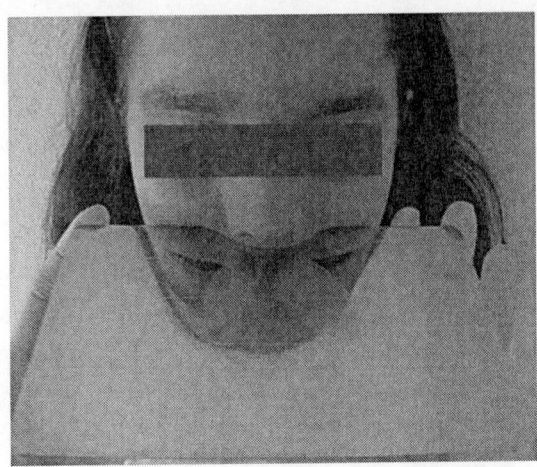

Figure 11. Breathing test – breathing condensation halo on the graded mirror.

The graded mirror test evaluates nasal air permeability and resistance by measuring the nasal airflow through the condensation of exhaled air on a metal plate, aiding in the identification of possible airway obstructions. In a study conducted by our group, it was found that most mouth breathing children produced a mirror condensation halo of less than 30 mm, which is considered low flow [7].

There may also be a decrease in masticatory muscle tone, making it even harder for the child to eat. This parameter can be evaluated through subjective tests. Another important factor to be observed in the evaluation is the alteration of the sense of smell, in case the child shows a deficit in gustatory perception and/or taste. Although speech plays a secondary role as to the basic functions of breathing, chewing and swallowing, it should not be neglected in the assessment. In mouth breathers, there is hyponasality or hypernasality during speech, due to dysfunctions of the soft palate, tongue posture and nasal aeration.

Altered phonemes occur when there are dysfunctions in the lips, tongue, velopharyngeal sphincter, swallowing, chewing movements, changes in dental occlusion or hypertrophic tonsils [42].

Postural features of the head, neck, shoulder, shoulder girdle, lumbar spine, dorsal and cervical spine, trunk and feet, at rest and while walking can be subjectively evaluated by goniometry and symmetography, or in a quantitative way through digital photogrammetry and stabilometry [43]. The subjective method assesses static alignment, inclinations, rotations of the head and spine (cervical, thoracic and lumbar) segments, shoulder, hip, knee and ankle joints, and foot positioning. The evaluation through digital photogrammetry, which quantitatively assesses postural asymmetries, combines digital photography with computer software for measuring horizontal and vertical angles and distances [44]. In the last few years, digital stabilometry has been often employed. It consists in an apparatus for optical three-dimensional (3D) detection of the morphology of the trunk, based on the principle of rastereography (grids of bright stripes) combined with triangulation algorithms. This technique evaluates vertebral curves by measuring the most relevant biomechanical and postural parameters, revealing alterations that jeopardize the spine in a sensitive and precise way [45].

As with the evaluation of mouth breathing, the clinical history of children with suspected OSA includes investigating the frequency of recurrent upper respiratory tract infections associated with breathing effort or mouth breathing itself. Also, a few specific issues regarding snoring and sleep are included in the investigation. Those related to snoring include frequency, intensity, and duration of snoring, and also if it culminates with breathing effort or even with breathing interruption (apnea) during sleep. Questions related to the child's sleep address the sleeping environment, sleep latency, sleep quality, sleeping position, movements during sleep, awakenings or micro-awakenings, sleepwalking, enuresis, napping frequency during the day and daytime sleepiness. In addition to these, issues surrounding the child's behavior are addressed, following evidence that OSA has some effect on mood [32, 33]. In this context, the following parameters are evaluated: lack of attention, hyperactivity, aggressiveness, poor school performance, emotional lability, language expression skills, visual perception and memory [46].

The physical examination should assess the pondero-statural situation, as the growth of children with OSA tends to be below what is expected, with malnutrition or obesity being often observed. These assessments are made by anthropometric measurements and analysis of nutritional status, with appropriate weight, height and body mass index scales for each age and gender. A thorough evaluation of the nasal and oral cavities should look for evidence of chronic obstruction of the UA such as hypertrophy of the palatine tonsils (laterolateral and anteroposterior diameters) and turbinates, as well as a long-face craniofacial shape, mandibular retrusion, high and constricted hard palate, lengthened soft palate and lip posture at rest.

Associated clinical conditions such as neurological diseases and genetic craniofacial syndromes should also be evaluated. It is important to include a cardiac evaluation to investigate signs suggestive of right overload (echocardiography is recommended) and systemic arterial hypertension. The presence of thoracic deformities such as *pectus excavatum* or thoracic asymmetry, which suggest increased long-term respiratory effort, should also be evaluated [30].

IMAGE DIAGNOSIS

Combined with the anamnesis and craniofacial clinical observations of individuals with suspected breathing disorders, radiographic evaluation is the first routine complementary exam. *Cavum* radiography is a lateral radiograph of the face; it does not, however, have any standards for head positioning and it shows distortions in the image size, making any measurement quite impossible. Therefore, it allows only a visual assessment of nasopharyngeal airway size, estimating adenoid hypertrophy [47].

LCR, on the other hand, is not only useful for assessing UA obstruction and pharyngeal dimensions, but is also the most effective method for assessing the skeletal pattern and growth direction of the face. It is more reliable than *cavum* radiography, for it presents the face and the UA image in a size very close to the real one. The image is obtained in a standardized manner, with the patient's head kept in a stable position and at a constant distance from the X-ray source by means of a cephalostat. LCR allows two-dimensional visualization and measurement of the UA, having been shown to be an important method for assessing adenoid obstruction, especially in children [48].

Nasofibroscopy is considered the gold standard for the diagnosis of adenoid hypertrophy. However, it is a difficult test for children, who generally do not accept a second intervention [5]. It consists in introducing an extremely thin, flexible optic fiber into each of the nasal cavities separately, for direct visualization of the nasal mucosa and the structures of the UA such as the nasal septum, inferior and middle turbinates and the adenoid. The resulting images can be video-recorded for further evaluation [49].

According to the international classification of sleep disorders – ICSD-3, a unified diagnosis based on signs and symptoms of pediatric OSA has been established. Only one of the following findings must be present: snoring, difficult/obstructed breathing or daytime consequences such as excessive sleepiness, hyperactivity, etc. [24]. However, one must keep in mind that the clinical history and physical examination are not sufficient to diagnose pediatric OSA. To confirm the diagnosis, it is necessary to prescribe polysomnography with overnight capnography [50, 51]. This test is considered the gold standard for diagnosis and treatment control in children. Preferably, polysomnography should be performed in an outpatient setting (hospital or clinic), where the child is monitored for a whole night by a specialized professional during spontaneous and nocturnal sleep. This noninvasive test monitors multiple physiological variables, i.e., electroencephalogram (EEG), right and left electrooculogram (EOG), bilateral submental and tibial electromyogram (EMG), nasal and oral airflow through oronasal pressure cannula and thermistor sensors, thoracic and abdominal respiratory effort by uncalibrated inductance plethysmography, oxyhemoglobin saturation (SpO_2) by pulse oximetry, snoring sensor (microphone) and bed position. In addition, pediatric polysomnography, unlike the adult one, has capnography as an exclusive parameter [50]. The diagnostic criteria for pediatric OSA by polysomnography differ from those of the adult in some parameters. It requires (1) one or more obstructive events (obstructive or mixed apnea or obstructive hypopnea) per hour of sleep or (2) obstructive hypoventilation defined by $PaCO_2 > 50$ mm Hg for more than 25% of the sleeping period, along with snoring, paradoxical thoracoabdominal movement (in handsaw – the abdomen moves outward while the chest moves inwards during inspiration), or a flattened nasal inspiratory pressure waveform, a polysomnographic signal that characterizes RERA [24]. On the other hand, in teenagers from 13 years of age onwards, polysomnography follows the same criteria used for adults, whose apnea and hypopnea index (AHI) should be greater than 5 events/h with oxyhemoglobin desaturation ≥3% or respiratory effort-related arousals per hour of sleep [52].

It must be stressed out that, regardless of it being the gold standard in the diagnosis of OSA, polysomnography is a complex, expensive test that makes its routine indication as a screening approach impossible. Many factors contribute to it not being performed in children quite so often: high cost, inconvenience for both parents and children in spending the night in the laboratory, and the relatively low number of sleep study centers with trained personnel specialized in pediatric sleep disorders. Still, even with all these limitations, polysomnography remains the most objective and accurate test for the diagnosis of pediatric OSA [51, 53].

As with adults, polysomnography tests conducted at home with portable equipment have occasionally been used in children. Other simplified diagnostic methods, such as video recording and overnight oximetry, have also been indicated despite their low specificity. However, they do not exclude the need for a polysomnography. Daytime polysomnography has been used, though it underestimates the presence and severity of OSA [51].

Based on the above, the medical and scientific communities have been trying to employ less expensive and faster diagnostic methods/techniques, in order to meet the high demand of individuals with impacting clinical symptoms of OSA who have not yet been diagnosed. Among such methods, LCR, cone beam computed tomography (CBCT) and magnetic resonance imaging have been considered for the identification and screening of children with suspected OSA. However, these also do not exclude the need for polysomnography as a definitive diagnosis [54].

CBCT is an imaging test that allows 3D visualization of the constricted UA region, in addition to its volumetric quantification. Compared to LCR, which is a 2D image, the main limitations of CBCT are still the high cost, higher radiation dose and lack of patient head standardization during acquisition, which may result in significant variability in the measurements [47].

On the other hand, LCR has been employed to identify UA obstructions and the degree of obstruction that can cause changes in facial bone growth [55, 56, 57]. In the 1980s, McNamara proposed that the nasopharyngeal width should be measured by LCR for the diagnosis of adenoid hypertrophy, defining the nasopharyngeal width as the shortest distance between a point at half of the posterior soft palate contour to the point closest to the posterior pharyngeal wall contour in the adenoid area (Figure 12). He found that the average distance of this line was of 12 mm for mixed dentition and 17.4 mm for adults of both sexes, considering that there was critical impairment of the airflow when this measurement was equal to or less than 5 mm.

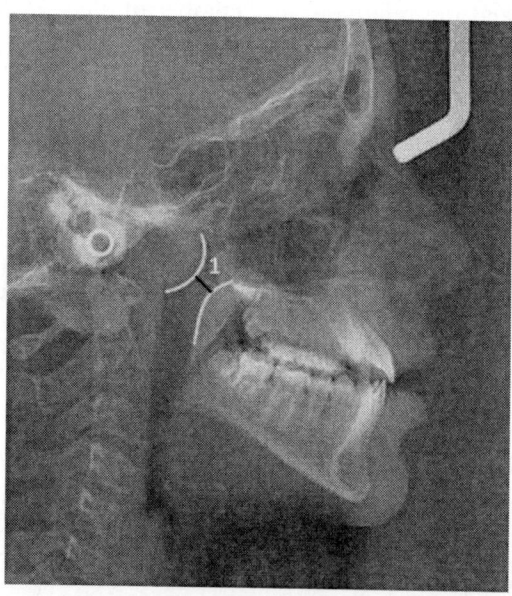

Figure 12. Lateral cephalometric radiograph (LCR) showing the (1) nasopharyngeal width measurement.

LCR has been validated as a reliable instrument for measuring the dimension of the nasopharynx and retropalatal regions, allowing the assessment of adenoid size, an important risk factor for the development of OSA in children [58, 59]. In a study conducted by our research group, it was found that children with decreased airway in the nasopharynx region (equal to or less than 5 mm) presented a tendency towards vertical growth, skeletal Class II malocclusion, increased oropharynx width (suggestive of hypertrophic palatine tonsils) and a significant increase in the length of the UA (Figure 13). Based on these results, we put forward that the increase in the UA length observed by LCR should be used to aid in the early diagnosis of pediatric OSA, working also as a screening step for children who need referrals for more specific exams such as polysomnography [60].

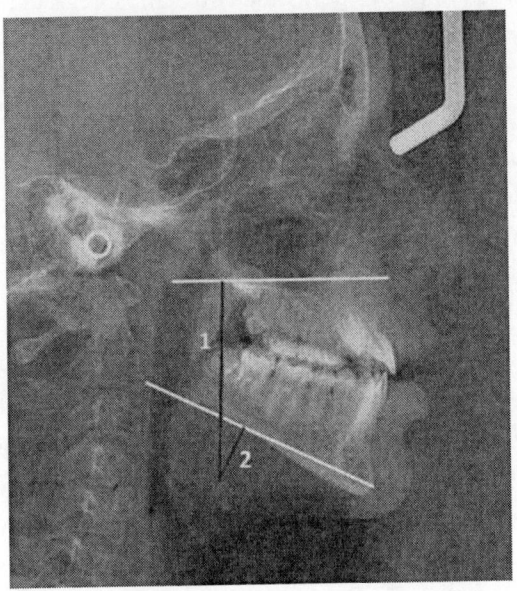

Figure 13. Main vertical upper airway (UA) measurements in the LCR. (1) UA vertical length from the posterior nasal spine to the hyoid bone. (2) Perpendicular distance between hyoid bone and lower edge of the mandible.

Therefore, the identification of risk factors for an early recognition of pediatric OSA may result in the development of treatments to eliminate the problems, or at the very least to decrease their impact on the lives of this population.

Treatment Options for Mouth Breathing and Pediatric Obstructive Sleep Apnea

In children who are not under life-threatening conditions, identifying and treating the causes that may contribute to the development of mouth breathing and OSA is a preventive measure, for sleep-related breathing disorders that remain undiagnosed or untreated in childhood may progress to severe apnea in adulthood. That is why the diagnosis and treatment of these disorders should be performed in an integrated manner by a multidisciplinary team [61].

Medicine is responsible for treating etiological agents and nasopharyngeal changes in a conservative or surgical way; Dentistry intervenes in osseo-myo-facial and dental arch disharmonies, correcting skeletal and dental alterations; Speech therapy is responsible for re-educating the structures and functions of the orofacial region, including the UA, adjusting muscle tonicity, mobility and posture of stomatognathic system structures; Physiotherapy intervenes in the acquisition of an ideal posture, creating new postural schemes, and in the rehabilitation of the respiratory muscles with stretching, strength and resistance exercises. When positive airway pressure (PAP) is prescribed, a physiotherapist adapts the mask, adjusts the ideal positive pressure for each child, and monitors the treatment to ensure proper adhesion to the use of the PAP device [62]. Besides those aforesaid fields, other specialties – oral-maxillofacial and head and neck surgeons, nutritionists, psychologists, physical educators, among others – can be involved in the treatment of mouth breathing and OSA. Some treatment alternatives may be conservative or surgical, depending on each case.

Regardless of the role played by each professional, they should all advise on the behavioral and habit alterations required for children with breathing disorders. Among these is weight loss, for a direct relationship between the reduction of OSA severity and weight loss has been well-established. The practice of physical exercise, in addition to facilitating weight loss, improves lung function, sleep quality and the child's quality of life, reducing symptoms associated to OSA. Along with physical activity, the adoption of healthy eating habits should also be recommended, under the guidance of a professional nutritionist. Finally, as fragmented sleep is an issue here, recommendations on that regard should also be made. Children with OSA should practice sleep hygiene, starting with the use of a comfortable mattress and a pillow that fills the shoulder-to-neck space, in order to promote spinal alignment; they should be instructed to keep bedtime regular; to do not use the bedroom to watch TV, read or study. They should also avoid the consumption of stimulants such as coffee, black tea, cola drinks, chocolate, among others, before bedtime.

The most common clinical and surgical treatment options for mouth breathing and OSA in children are very similar (Figure 14).

Treatment options for pediatric OSA	
Clinical management	Allergic rhinitis treatment Weight loss (for obese children) Continuous positive airway pressure (CPAP or BiLevel) when recommended Orthodontics and dentofacial orthopedics treatment
Surgical treatment	Adenotonsillectomy Orthognathic surgeries (for children with craniofacial malformations) Tracheostomy (indicated in some cases)

Figure 14. Treatment options for pediatric OSA.

The clinical management of allergic rhinitis and the surgical removal of the adenoid and palatine tonsils are the most often employed approaches.

Regarding allergic rhinitis, the treatment may be etiological or symptomatic, depending on the intensity of the reactions and their persistence over time. The etiological treatment consists in: 1. allergen suppression – which consists in identifying the allergen and its distribution and, if possible, avoiding it; 2. immunotherapy – which employs subcutaneous injections with increasing amounts of allergens. The symptomatic treatment consists in the administration of various nasal or systemic drugs [38, 63].

In some instances, the hypertrophy of lymphoid tissues, particularly the adenoid and palatine tonsils, can be reduced by means of pharmacological therapy [61]. However, in those cases in which hypertrophy is causing airway obstruction and consequent deformation of the facial growth, surgical removal should be considered. Thus, adenoidectomy and tonsillectomy are the most common surgical procedures performed in children. Not that long ago, these surgeries used to be recommended only for cases of recurrent tonsillitis, which are now much less frequent thanks to advances in antibiotic therapy. On the other hand, surgeries for the hypertrophy of adenoid and palatine tonsils promote a proven gain in the child's quality of life [2]. All professionals involved in the child's care must be aware of the benefits of adenotonsillectomy, in order not to make the family insecure about the procedure.

The recognition of the signs and symptoms of OSA in children by all medical areas has brought faster diagnosis and treatment. It is important that the treatment be conducted at a growing age, in order to minimize the consequent skeletal alterations of the face and the comorbidities that alter the child's body, intellectual and emotional development. Nevertheless, the surgical indication cannot be established solely on the basis of clinical history and physical examination, but must also consider airway dynamics during sleep. It is worthy of note that breathing disorders are exacerbated or may appear only during sleep, thus the need for a detailed clinical history and an evaluation of diurnal and nocturnal symptoms.

The benefits achieved by orthodontic and facial orthopedic treatments are more stable long-term when the respiratory function is normalized, thus the concern of dentistry with keeping the UA unobstructed and nose breathing following the removal of the obstruction. To begin with, the infant patient with obstructive mouth breathing should be referred to the otolaryngologist, who evaluates the best way to clear the UA, either by medication or surgery. Following the reduction of the obstruction, awareness and training are performed to ensure that those who acquired the habit of breathing through the mouth can do so again through the nose. This training can be done prior to or concomitantly with orthodontic treatment, in order to achieve long-term stability of the results. Patients receive guidance on lip sealing, tongue posture at rest, swallowing and phonation without tongue interposition. They are then encouraged to do the daily lip-sealing exercise previously recommended in the "Lip sealing routine to eliminate the habit of mouth breathing" (Figure 10), which consists in sealing the mouth with tape for an increasing amount of time each day, according to one's ability, progressively increasing the time until the person can breathe only through the nose for at least two consecutive hours. Parents should ensure that this training is performed daily, when their child's attention is focused on tasks that are independent of mouth use, i.e., playing games, watching television, etc. [8]. The input of a speech therapist is most welcome in these cases, in order to restore muscle tonicity and the balance between the inner and outer muscles of the mouth.

Orthodontics and facial orthopedics employed in the treatment of mouth breathing and OSA in children aim to increase the internal buccal space. The goal is the interception and correction of skeletal and dental disharmonies that affect the normal growth and development of the face and UA, mainly triggered by untreated breathing problems. Because mouth breathing children may develop different types of dental and skeletal alterations, depending on the muscle compensations that result from the nasal airway obstruction [3, 4], orthodontic devices are prescribed with the primary purposes of harmonizing the bony bases, providing greater breadth of the oral and nasal spaces, and balancing form and function. The most commonly used orthodontic and facial orthopedic treatments for this purpose are rapid maxillary expansion (RME), closure of the anterior open bite, maxillary protraction, and mandible advancement. Treatments may also include the removal of deleterious oral habits, controlling of the vertical dimension, increasing the masticatory area by opening spaces and replacing missing teeth, harmonizing the dental arches to enable maxillary and/or mandibular surgical advancements, among others that may be related to breathing disorders.

Skeletal and dental malocclusions affecting children between 3 and 12 years of age should be treated during deciduous and mixed dentition, with the exception of mandibular growth deficiency problems, which are most effective when treated at the onset of permanent dentition during the pubertal growth spurt. Treatments requiring orthognathic surgery should generally be postponed to the end of the growth phase. Malocclusions can occur on all three facial axes: transverse, vertical and anteroposterior. The most common malocclusions in each axis are: 1. Constricted maxilla, which is the narrowing of the hard palate on the transverse axis that may lead to posterior crossbite. It should be treated by opening the midpalatal suture with rapid maxillary expansion appliances; 2. Anterior open bite, which is the lack of contact between the upper and lower anterior teeth on the vertical axis. It should be treated by removing or controlling the cause (UA obstruction, deleterious oral habits, divergent growth of facial bones) and with devices to reestablish dental occlusion; 3. Maxillary retrusion or mandibular retrusion, which is the deficiency in the growth of the middle third of the face (maxilla) or mandible in the anteroposterior axis. It should be treated with devices that promote maxillary protraction or mandibular advancement.

A systematic review and meta-analysis conducted in 2016 proved the effectiveness of rapid maxillary expansion and orthopedic mandibular advancement in the treatment of snoring and pediatric OSA [64].

Maxillary expansion is used to correct maxillary transverse deficiency, consisting in the painless opening of the midpalatal suture (Figure 15). An appliance containing an expander screw is fixed to the teeth, thus a unique block is formed between teeth, bones and the appliance itself. Each activation of the screw transmits to the teeth a heavy tension that inhibits their movement. This tension is then transmitted to the facial sutures, especially to the midpalatal suture, producing a distraction that stimulates bone neoformation. In children, the midpalatal suture is not yet consolidated, which allows its opening with different models of expansion devices, providing they offer proper anchorage to the supporting teeth. Maxillary expansion can be done rapidly, with the expanders attached to the supporting teeth. It can also be done slowly with removable expanders, although these will make a predominantly dentoalveolar expansion rather than at the midpalatal suture. Fixed expanders are usually made of stainless-steel bands welded to the expander screw, being attached to the teeth at four points. But they can also be made of acrylic resin directly in plaster model and be cemented to the teeth (Figure 16B), which avoids the adaptation of bands in very young children, or in those expulsive, little erupted teeth.

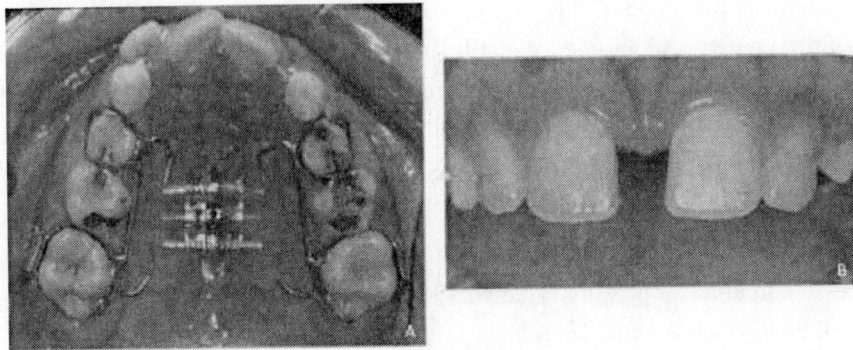

Figure 15. A-B. (A) Haas-type fixed expander for rapid maxillary expansion. (B) Opening of the midpalatal suture with separation of the upper central incisors.

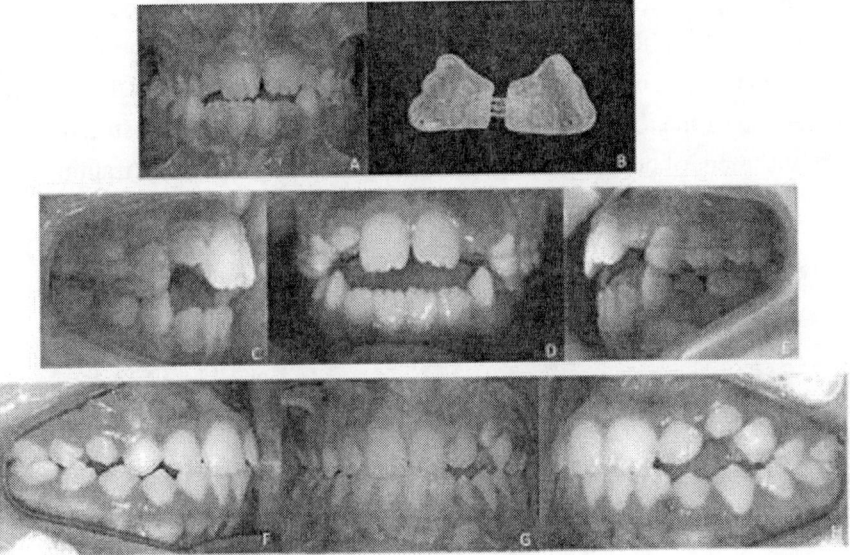

Figure 16. A-H. Treatment of posterior crossbite and maxillary constriction with the encapsulated expander. (A) Initial malocclusion. (B) Encapsulated expander, (C-D-E) Encapsulated expander cemented to the teeth. (F-G-H) After the intervention.

Rapid maxillary expansion has been put forward as an effective treatment for pediatric OSA. A systematic review and meta-analysis conducted in 2017 found a reduction in AHI and improved oxygen saturation in children with OSA. The authors noted that the results were better in children with previous adenotonsillectomy or in those with small tonsils than in those with large tonsils [65]. Our recommendation is that the UA should be unobstructed in advance to ensure long-term results. The reason for that is quite plain: the tongue in its normal position, touching the palate during swallowing and at rest, is the main responsible for the normal palate shape. The presence of hypertrophied tonsils forces the tongue to assume an altered, lower and anterior posture. That way it does not continually shape the palate and, consequently, enables relapses of constricted maxilla.

The correction of skeletal disharmony in the transverse dimension of the face should always be performed first, as vertical and anteroposterior disharmonies almost always present some degree of constricted maxilla, thus benefiting from its correction. Figure 17A-F shows the correction of anterior open bite by an appliance that simultaneously performs the transverse expansion of the maxilla and the prevention of the anterior projection of the tongue. All etiological factors, such as UA obstruction, re-establishment of nose breathing, lip sealing and tongue posture training, had been previously dealt with.

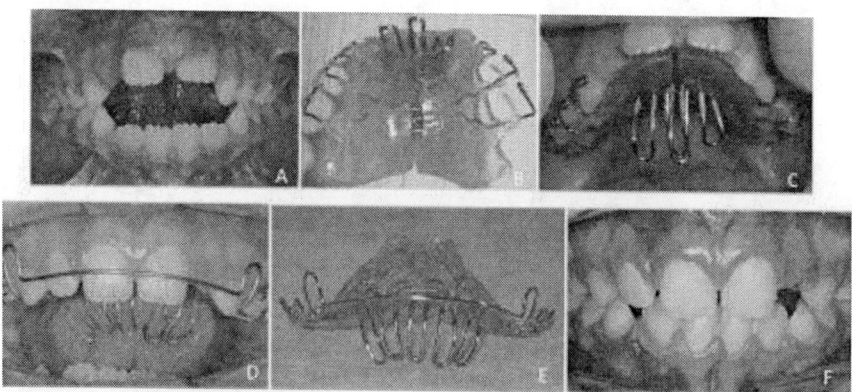

Figure 17. A-F. Treatment of anterior open bite. (A) Initial malocclusion. (B-C) Removable appliance with expander and curtain-shape palatal crib. (D-E-F) After jaw expansion, closing of the bite with palatal crib.

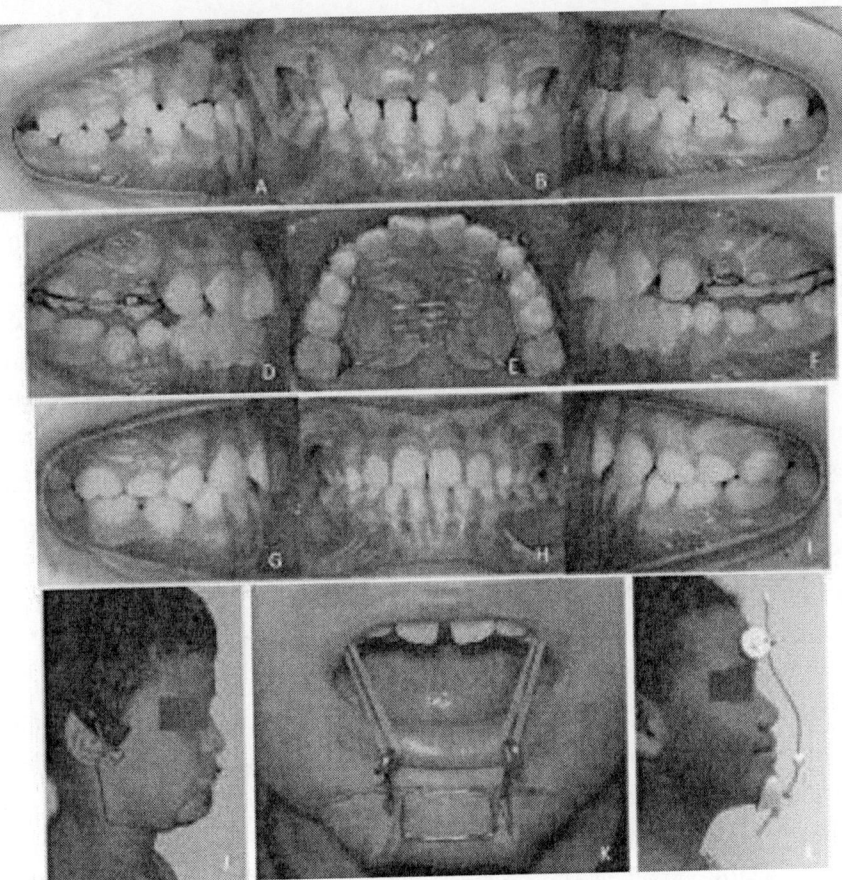

Figure 18. A-L. Treatment of maxillary retrusion with a facial mask. (A-B-C) Initial malocclusion. (D-E-F) The Haas-type modified expander with hooks maintains the maxilla as a single bone. (D e F) Lower inclined plane assists in the correction of anterior crossbite (G-H-I) Occlusion after the intervention. (J-K) Elastics and a facial mask promote maxillary protraction. (L) Facial mask with chin and forehead support.

Maxillary retrusion is a deficiency in the growth of the middle third of the face that impacts the UA, promoting the development of pediatric OSA. Facial orthopedic treatment of this skeletal disharmony involves the opening of the anteroposterior sutures of the maxillary complex, especially the zygomaticomaxillary, frontomaxillary, and pterygoid-palatine sutures, and forwarding the maxilla. For that are employed an intraoral device that forms a single block with maxillary teeth and bones (usually the maxillary expansion device itself, with additional hooks), and an extraoral device that allows the maxillary complex to be pulled anteriorly through elastic bands. Figure 18 A-K shows the treatment of maxillary retrusion by means of the expander with hooks in the region of the upper canines, where the elastics that make the anterior traction of the maxilla – which is held by an extraoral device (facial mask) with chin and skull supports – are adapted. Several types of facial mask can be used for this purpose, the most usual ones being those with chin and forehead supports (Figure 18L). Additional intraoral devices may be employed to facilitate forward movement, such as the fixed lower inclined plane, which is used to ease the correction of anterior crossbite. The treatment depends on patient compliance and should be introduced before age 10 [66]. Long-term stability falls around 70% to 75%, depending not only on maxillary growth, but also on the degree and direction of mandibular growth, which will only reach its maximum point at puberty [66]. Maxillary protraction promotes increased UA volume [67] and nasopharyngeal dimension [68, 69], minimizing the severity of a future orthognathic surgery if that ever comes to be necessary.

Mandibular retrusion is the deficiency in mandibular growth that particularly affects OSA patients. This skeletal deficiency is highly influenced by genetics and should not be treated in the early stages of early deciduous or mixed dentition, nor wait for adulthood. The treatment of this problem should be performed at the pubertal growth spurt, by the end of mixed dentition, when the greatest gains in mandibular growth can be obtained. Hand and wrist radiographs or the analysis of cervical vertebrae maturation in the LCR may be indicative of when it would be best to start treatment. Several types of removable or fixed appliances can be used to protrude the growing child's mandible, with fixed ones being more effective than removable ones. Figure 19 A-I shows the treatment of mandibular retrusion with the Herbst appliance, which provides continuous mandibular protrusion. The appliance is installed bilaterally in the mandible and supported on the upper teeth. In order to prevent the latter from moving, the maxilla must be anchored through an intraoral device – usually the maxillary expander itself – that forms a single block with maxillary teeth and bones. The Herbst appliance is adjustable and does not stop the mandible from moving laterally. Smaller, more comfortable Herbst appliances are currently available (Figure 19J). The treatment significantly increases the oropharynx and laryngopharynx [70, 71, 72], reducing the obstructive AHI in children [73, 74]. It also increases oxygen saturation, along with having few side effects, good acceptability and excellent cost-effectiveness compared to the continuous positive airway pressure (CPAP) device [74]. Long-term studies reveal optimal stability of the mandibular advancement treatment with Herbst appliance [75, 76].

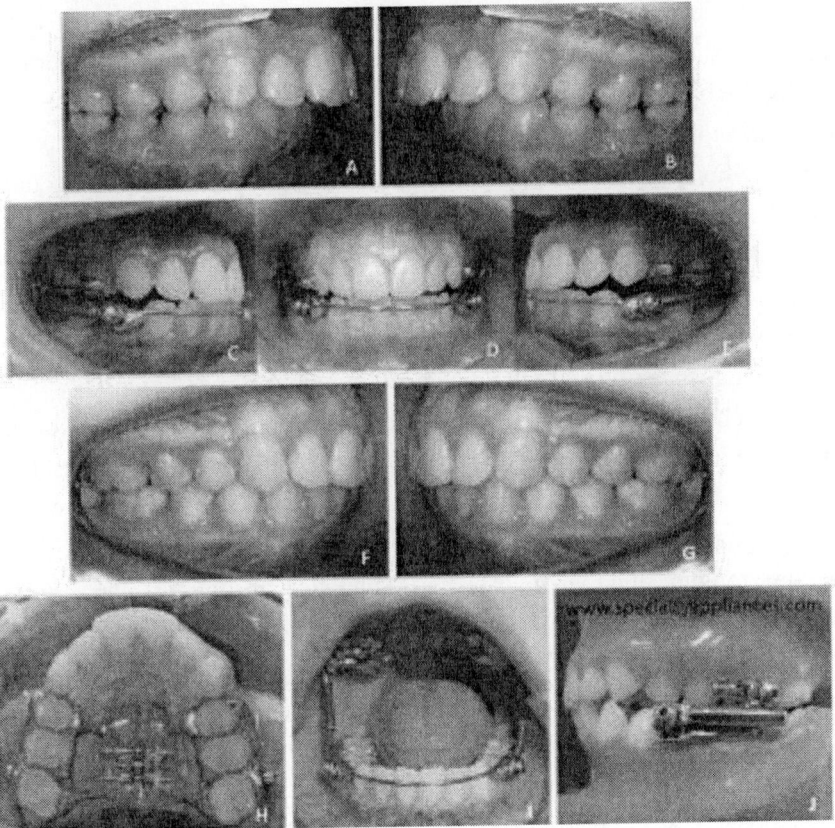

Figure 19. A-J. Treatment of mandibular retrusion with the Herbst appliance for mandibular advancement. (A-B) Initial malocclusion. (C-D-E) Devices installed with mandibular advancement. (F-G) Final occlusion. (H) The maxilla is supported by a Haas-type expander that holds (I) the Herbst appliance. (J) Smaller and more comfortable type of Herbst appliance for mandibular advancement (source: Miniscope® - Specialty Appliances Ortho Lab).

Speech therapy intervention in mouth breathing and pediatric OSA consists, at first, of raising the awareness of children and their families about the damage caused by mouth breathing. The functioning of the respiratory system and the importance of proper breathing should also be made clear, as well as the guidance of family members as to ways not to aggravate the craniofacial alterations of the child. Speech therapy is also concerned with the re-establishment of nasal breathing, in which the child learns to use her nose again through continuous training, not only in therapy but also at home, in order to obtain the best results [77]. The stimuli to reinforce the use of the nasal cavity are made by means of a graded mirror (biofeedback therapy), and by the blindfolded detection of different odors. For these interventions the child should keep the lips sealed.

Specific isometric and isotonic exercises should be performed in order to enhance muscle tonicity and improve the posture of the phono-articulatory organs. These exercises strengthen the muscles of the lips and cheeks, lengthen the upper lip filter, and relax the mental muscle, improving not only breathing but also other stomatognathic functions such as chewing, swallowing, speaking and the voice itself, which may be altered.

Speech therapy treatment through myofunctional therapy also consists in improving body posture and performing basic isometric and isotonic exercises, in order to improve the mobility and strength of the stomatognathic system muscles, with emphasis on the posterior musculature of the tongue and velopharyngeal sphincter. Isometric and isotonic myofunctional exercises are performed in the soft palate regions to promote the elevation of the soft palate, uvula and palatoglossal arch muscles, in order to open space between palate and tongue. In the face, these exercises consist in facial mimics, involving the orbicular muscle of the mouth, the buccinator, zygomatic major and minor muscles, upper lip and angle elevators, lateral and medial pterygoid muscles. The tongue is also involved, recruiting and contracting the genioglossus, hyoglossus, styloglossus, superior and inferior longitudinal, palatoglossus and suprahyoid muscles. One could, for instance, work on the sustained protrusion and snapping of the tongue, and brushing the tongue in the opposite direction from front to back while trying to keep it behind the lower teeth, which works both intrinsic and extrinsic muscles and enables a new, more superior tongue position at rest (Figure 20).

As the mouth breather presents breathing, postural and structural problems, the planning of the physical therapy treatment must be careful. One should assess the advantages of treating all the alterations at the same time over fragmenting them first. Based on this assumption, physical therapy can involve techniques ranging from the most conventional to the most specific ones, such as manual therapy.

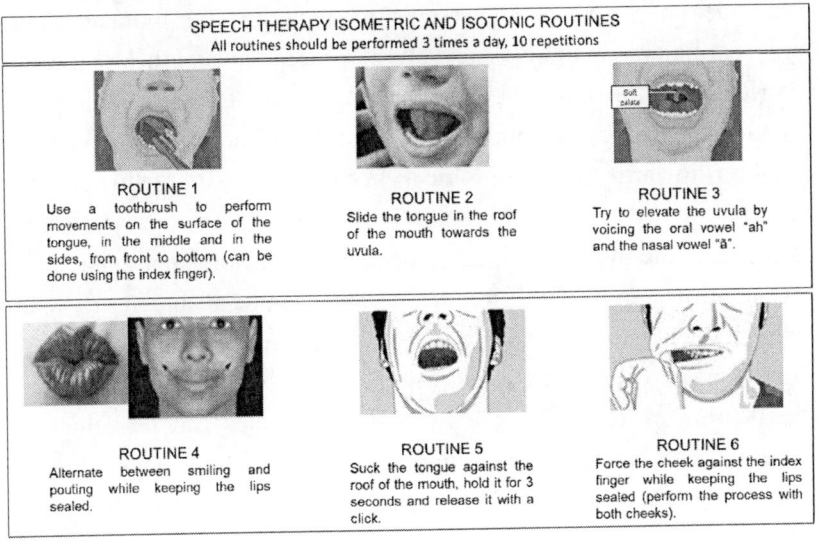

Figure 20. Speech therapy isometric and isotonic routines.

Some of the conventional treatments that can be used are electrotherapy, massage therapy and kinesiotherapy. The latter is the most suitable one, for it reorganizes muscle harmony through relaxation, stretching and strengthening.

Manual therapy techniques comprise treatments that involve stretching muscle or myofascial chains of children with breathing disorders, using methods such as global postural reeducation (GPR), global stretching (active global stretching/iso-stretching), postural reprogramming or posturology, and the muscle and articular chain method [78]. GPR consists in rebalancing the myofascial tensions that may be responsible for joint overload, by acting on the stretching of contracted or retracted antigravity muscles within different static muscle chains [79]. Global stretching is indicated after GPR, in order to continue the stretching of muscles that have remained shortened and still cause imbalances in the body. The postural reprogramming method is used to reprogram the tonic-postural system, involving maneuvers that are employed to understand and circumscribe altered postural inputs, aiming at global postural reprogramming at the central nervous system level. However, the connective tissue must be taken into consideration, for fascial structures can be shortened around any type of muscle [78].

In order to correct or adjust posture, including the thoracic changes (thorax carinatum or thorax excavatum) present in mouth breathing and pediatric OSA, the physical therapy program is focused on improving respiratory mechanics. Respiratory physical therapy aims to lead pulmonary ventilation towards a physiological standard, i.e., with lower energy expenditure by the child. Through respiratory kinesiotherapy, physical therapy helps the mouth breather to become a nose-breather again, as well as to control the rhythm, frequency and depth of breathing. During breathing, the inspiratory and expiratory movements made by the thorax and abdomen enable the work and awareness of the breathing movements. Strengthening exercises for the respiratory muscles can be achieved by counter-resisted breathing, breathing against a weight, the physiotherapist's hand, the divan or bed itself, as well as through sustained breathing, fractional breathing, prolonged and resisted expiration. While these kinesiotherapy resources are helpful, respiratory enhancers such as Threshold®, Triflo®, and Voldyne® are more effective when it comes to strength gain and respiratory muscle endurance. The thoracoabdominal rebalancing technique can be used in the treatment of breathing disorders and is based on muscle and myofascial massages, stretching and strengthening of accessory respiratory muscles, facilitation and strengthening of the diaphragm, restructuring of normal articular positioning, tactile and proprioceptive stimulation.

When is recommended that a child with OSA use positive airway pressure (PAP) after polysomnographic diagnosis, the treatment can be performed using two types of devices: CPAP (Continuous Positive Airway

Pressure), which is indicated in most cases, and the Bilevel Positive Airway Pressure to maintain two levels of pressure, which is recommended in cases of obesity hypoventilation syndrome, congenital alveolar hypoventilation syndrome (Ondine syndrome), and for patients with associated lung diseases [80, 81].

The PAP device may be of fixed pressure or automatic. In the former, one sets the pressure determined by the titration polysomnography. In automatic devices, the pressure can be set within a range from 4 to 20 cm H_2O. The devices have a ramp mode that allows a gradual pressure gain until the stipulated pressure is reached. A flexible tube connects the device to a mask (nasal, oronasal or facial), which is adapted to the child's face by means of elastic straps. When the appliance is turned on, it releases a pressure airflow that is directed to the child's UA, being then transmitted to the internal lumen of the pharynx. The resulting expansion of the lumen ensures pharyngeal patency, preventing its collapse [80]. From the first night of PAP use, apnea and snoring disappear and oxyhemoglobin saturation is normalized. Adaptation to the device is similar for children and adults. First, the child and her family members are made aware of the clinical implications of OSA and the benefits that PAP brings to the child's health and quality of life, if used correctly. Next, a step-by-step mask installation and connection to the device takes place. The appliance should be handled by the child and family members in the on and off modes, and additional information regarding cleaning and periodic filter change should be made available.

Individualized masks must be chosen in order to ensure an ideal adaptation [82]. Nasal masks should be tried first, for they have smaller area of contact with the face, are more comfortable, require less pressure, suffer less leakage and are more economically viable, being thus related to a better adherence of children to the treatment [80]. In addition, for each type of mask there is a variety of designs, sizes and materials, meeting the different needs of the population. The selected mask is attached to the child's face by means of snap-in frames whose straps are attached to the head. To prevent phobia from taking place, as soon as the mask is adapted to the face, the child is told to breathe gently for a certain period, being asked as to feeling comfortable during the process. The mask is then attached to the tube, and the tube to the PAP device. During the adaptation period, the presence of leaks – in different body positions – should be evaluated and, if they do occur, adjustments should be made until the leaking is completely abolished. The child remains for about an hour with the device turned on, during which she will be instructed to make decubitus changes in order to check if the mask stays put, to make sure there will be no air leakage in any of these positions. At the end of this period, the child and her family member perform the entire mask and appliance installation procedure again under the supervision of the physical therapist. At the end of the procedure, a written script with all the steps to be replicated before the child sleeps is given to the family member.

CONCLUSION

It is no longer possible to deny the influence of mouth breathing on the onset of pediatric OSA. The truth is, there is no better treatment than prevention. Thus, children with airway obstruction should be identified and treated to prevent the physiological need for breathing through the mouth from becoming a habit of mouth breathing. Those who have acquired the habit of mouth breathing must be re-educated to breathe again through the nose. Craniofacial and postural changes that may be present should be acknowledged and corrected during the growth phase. Only in this way can the progression to more severe sleep-disordered breathing in adulthood be prevented.

REFERENCES

[1] Sisniega, Carlos and Umakanth Katwa. 2019. "Children with upper airway dysfunction: at risk of obstructive sleep apnea." *J Child Sci.* 9:e59–e67. https://doi:10.1055/s-0039-1688956.

[2] Guilleminault, Christian and Yu-Shu Huang. 2018. "From oral facial dysfunction to dysmorphism and the onset of pediatric OSA." *Sleep Medicine Reviews.* 40: 203-14. http://dx.doi:10.1016/j.smrv.2017.06.008. Epub 2017 Jul 6.

[3] Harvold, Egil P, Tomer, BS, Vargervik, K, Chierici, G. 1981. "Primate experiments on oral respiration." *Am J Orthod.* 79(4):359-72. https://doi.org/10.1016/0002-9416(81)90379-1.

[4] Vargervik Karin, Miller, AJ, Chierici, G, Harvold, E, Tomer, BS. 1984. "Morphologic response to changes in neuromuscular patterns experimentally induced by altered modes of respiration." *Am J Orthod.* 85(2):115-24. https://doi.org/10.1016/0002-9416(84)90003-4.

[5] Di Vece, Luca, Doldo, T, Faleri, G, Picciotti, M, Salerni, L, Ugolini, A, Goracci, C. 2018. "Rhinofibroscopic and rhinomanometric evaluation of patients with maxillary contraction treated with rapid maxillary expansion. A prospective pilot study." *J Clin Pediatr Dent.* 42(1):27-31. https://doi.org/10.17796/1053-4628-42.1.5.

[6] Bozzini, Maria FR and Di Francesco RC. 2016. "Managing obstructive sleep apnoea in children: the role of craniofacial morphology." *Clinics.* 1,71(11): 664-66. http://doi.org/10.6061/clinics/2016(11)08.

[7] Pacheco, M Christina T, Fiorott, BS, Finck, NS, Araujo, MTM. 2015a. "Craniofacial changes and symptoms of sleep-disordered breathing in healthy children." *Dental Press J Orthod.* 20:80-7. http://doi:10.1590/2176-9451.20.3.080-087.oar.

[8] Pacheco, M Christina T, Casagrande, CF, Teixeira, LP, Finck, NS, Araújo, MTM. 2015b. "Guidelines proposal for clinical recognition of mouth breathing children." *Dental Press J Orthod.* 20:39-44. http://doi:10.1590/2176-9451.20.4.039-044.oar.

[9] Abreu, Rubens R, Rocha, RL, Lamounier, JA, Guerra, AFM. 2008. "Etiology, clinical manifestations and concurrent findings in mouth-breathing children." *J Pediatr.* 84(6):529-35. https://doi.org/10.1590/S0021-75572008000700010

[10] Araújo, Maria TM and M Christina T Pacheco. 2018. "*Distúrbios Respiratórios na Infância: da respiração oral à apneia obstrutiva do sono.*" (Childhood Breathing Disorders: from mouth breathing to

obstructive sleep apnea) Vitória: UFES, 1-96. ISBN: 978-85-924668-0-0. http://www.odontologia.ufes.br/sites/odontologia.ufes.br/files/field/anexo/livro_disturbios_respiratorios_na_infancia_-mestrado.pdf

[11] Neiva, Patricia D, Kirkwood, RN, Godinho R. 2009. "Orientation and position of head posture, scapula and thoracic spine in mouth-breathing children." *Int J Pediatr Otorhinolaryngol.* 73(2):227-36. https://doi.org/10.1016/j.ijporl.2008.10.006.

[12] Cuccia, Antonio M, Lotti, M, Caradonna, D. 2008. "Oral breathing and head posture." *Angle Orthod.* 78(1):77-82. https://doi.org/10.2319/011507-18.1.

[13] Okuro, Renata T, Morcillo, AM, Sakano, E, Schivinski, CIS, Ribeiro, MAGO, Ribeiro JD. 2011. "Exercise capacity, respiratory mechanics and posture in mouth breathers." *Braz J Otorhinolaryngol.* 77(5):656-62. http://dx.doi.org/10.1590/S1808-86942011000500020.

[14] Corrêa, Eliane CR and Fausto Bérzin. 2004. "Temporomandibular disorder and dysfunctional breathing." *Braz J Oral Sci.* 3:498-502. https://doi.org/10.20396/bjos.v3i10.8641760.

[15] Austin, David G. 2010. "Introduction to a postural education and exercise program in sleep medicine." *Sleep Med Clin.* 5(1):115-29. https://doi.org/10.1016/j.jsmc.2009.11.002.

[16] Armijo-Olivo, Susan, Rappoport, K, Fuentes, J, GadottI, I, Major, PW, Warren, S, Thie, NM, Magee, DJ. 2011. "Head and cervical posture in patients with temporomandibular disorders." *J Orofac Pain.* 25(3):199-209.

[17] Finck, Nathalia S, Santos Neto, ET, Araújo, MTM, Pacheco, MCT. 2015. Alterações craniofaciais, posturais e temporomandibulares associadas à respiração bucal em escolares de 7 a 13 anos. (Craniofacial, postural and temporomandibular changes associated with mouth breathing in schoolchildren aged 7-13). *Rev Bras Pesq Saúde/Brazilian Journal of Health Research.* 17(4): 38-47.

[18] Ribeiro, Andressa F, Morosini, LM, Finck, NS, Pacheco, MCT, Araújo, MTM. 2016. "Associação entre as adaptações da articulação temporomandibular e a qualidade de vida de escolares respiradores

bucais." (Association between the adaptations of the TMJ and life quality in school-age mouth-breathers). *Fisioter Bras.* 17(4):321-34.

[19] Yi, Liu C, Jardim, JR, Inoue, DP, Pignatari, SS. 2008. "The relationship between excursion of the diaphragm and curvatures of the spinal column in mouth breathing children." *J Pediatr.* 84(2):171-7. http://dx.doi.org/10.2223/JPED.1771.

[20] Silveira, Waleska, Mello, FCQ, Guimarães, FS, Menezes, SLS. 2010. "Postural alterations and pulmonary function of mouth-breathing children." *Braz J Otorhinolaryngol.* 76(6):683-86.

[21] Uhlig, Suélen E, Marchesi, LM, Duarte, H, Araújo, MTM. 2015. "Association between respiratory and postural adaptations and self-perception of school-aged children with mouth breathing in relation to their quality of life." *Braz J Phys Ther.* 19(3):201-10. http://dx.doi.org/10.1590/bjpt-rbf.2014.0087.

[22] Fitzpatrick, Michael F, McLean, H, Urton, AM, Tan, A, O'Donnell, D, Driver, HS. 2003. "Effect of nasal or oral breathing route on upper airway resistance during sleep." *Eur Respir J.* 22:827–32. http://doi.org/10.1183/09031936.03.00047903.

[23] Koutsourelakis, Ioannis, Vagiakis, E, Roussos, C, Zakynthinos, S. 2006. "Obstructive sleep apnoea and oral breathing in patients free of nasal obstruction." *Eur Respir J.* 28:1222–28. https://doi.org/10.1183/09031936.00058406

[24] Sateia, Michael J. 2014. "International classification of sleep disorders-third edition: highlights and modifications." *Chest.* 146(5):1387-94. doi: 10.1378/chest.14-0970. https://doi.org/10.1378/chest.14-0970.

[25] Sinha, Deepti and Christian Guilleminault. 2010. "Sleep disordered breathing in children." *Indian J Med Res.* 131:311-20.

[26] Redline, Susan, Tishler, PV, Schluchter, M, Aylor, J, Clark, K, Graham, G. 1999. "Risk factor for sleep-disordered breathing in children: associations with obesity, race and respiratory problems." *Am J Respir Crit Care Med* 159(5):1527-32. https://doi.org/10.1164/ajrccm.159.5.9809079.

[27] Izu, Suemy C, Itamoto, CH, Pradella-Hallinan, M, Pizarro, GU, Tufik, S, Pignatari, S, Fujita, RR. 2010. "Obstructive sleep apnea syndrome (OSAS) in mouth breathing children." *Braz J Otorhinolaryngol.* 76(5):552-6.

[28] Marcus, Carole, Chapman, D, Ward, S. 2002. "Clinical practice guideline: Diagnosis and management of childhood obstructive sleep apnea syndrome." *Pediatrics.* 109(4) 704-12. https://doi.org/10.1542/peds.2012-1671. Epub 2012 Aug 27

[29] Lumeng, Julie C and Chervin, RD. 2008. "Epidemiology of pediatric obstructive sleep apnea." *Proc Am Thorac Soc.* 5(2):242-52. https://doi.org/10.1513/pats.200708-135MG

[30] Kaditis, Athanasios G, Kaditis, AG, Alonso Alvarez, ML, Boudewyns, A, Alexopoulos, EI, Ersu, R, Joosten, K, Larramona, H, Miano, S, Narang, I, Trang, H, Tsaoussoglou, M, Vandenbussche, N, Villa, MP, Van Waardenburg, D, Weber, S, Verhulst, S. 2016. "Obstructive sleep disordered breathing in 2-to 18-year-old children: diagnosis and management." *Eur Respir J.* 47(1):69-94. https://doi.org/10.1183/13993003.00385-2015

[31] Amin, Raouf S, Kimball, TR, Kalra, M, Jeffries, JL, Carroll, JL, Bean, JA, Witt, SA, Glascock, BJ, Daniels, SR. 2005. "Left ventricular function in children with sleep-disordered breathing." *Am J Cardiol.* 95(6):801-4. https://doi.org/10.1016/j.amjcard.2004.11.044.

[32] Beebe, Dean W. 2006. "Neurobehavioral morbidity associated with disordered breathing during sleep in children: a comprehensive review." *Sleep.* 29(9):1115-34. https://doi.org/10.1093/sleep/29.9.1115.

[33] Hamasaki Uema, Sandra F, NagataPignatari, SS, Fujita, RR, Moreira, GA, Pradella-Hallinan, M, Weckx, L. 2007. "Assessment of cognitive learning function in children with obstructive sleep breathing disorders." *Braz J Otorhinolaryngol.* 73(3):315-20. https://doi.org/10.1016/S1808-8694(15)30074-4.

[34] Row, Barry W, Liu, R, Xu, W, Kheirandish, L, Gozal, D. 2003. "Intermittent hypoxia is associated with oxidative stress and spatial

learning deficits in the rat." *Am J Respir Crit Care Med.* 167(11):1548-53. https://doi.org/10.1164/rccm.200209-1050OC.

[35] Bass, Joel L, Corwin, M, Gozal, D, Moore, C, Nishida, H, Parker, S., Schonwald, A, Wilker, R E, Stehle, S, Kinane, T B. 2004. "The effect of chronic or intermittent hypoxia on cognition in childhood: a review of the evidence." *Pediatrics.* 114(3):805-16. https://doi.org/10.1542/peds.2004-0227

[36] Carvalho, Luciane B, Prado, LB, Silva, L, Almeida, MM, Silva, TA, Vieira, CM, Atallah, AN, Prado, GF. 2004. "Cognitive dysfunction in children with sleep disorders." *Arq Neuro-Psiquiatr.* 62(2A):212-6. http://dx.doi.org/10.1590/S0004-282X2004000200004.

[37] Kikuchi, Makoto. 2005. "Orthodontic treatment in children to prevent sleep-disordered breathing in adulthood." *Sleep Breath.* 9:146–158. https://doi.org/10.1007/s11325-005-0028-8.

[38] Ibiapina, Cássio da C, Sarinho, ESC, Camargos, PAM, de Andrade, CR, Filho, AASC. 2008. "Allergic rhinitis: epidemiological aspects, diagnosis and treatment." *J Bras Pneumol.* 34(4):230-40. http://dx.doi.org/10.1590/S1806-37132008000400008.

[39] Brodsky, Linda. 1989. "Modern assessment of tonsils and adenoid." *Pediatric Clin North Am.* 36:1551-69. https://doi.org/10.1016/S0031-3955(16)36806-7.

[40] Friedman, Michael, Tanyeri, H, La Rosa, M, Landsberg, R, Vaidyanathan, K, Pieri, S, Caldarelli, D. 1999. "Clinical predictors of obstructive sleep apnea." *Laryngoscope.* 109(12):1901-7. https://doi.org/10.1097/00005537-199912000-00002.

[41] Proffit, WR, Fields, HW, Larson, B, Sarver, DM. 2018. *"Contemporary Orthodontics."* 6th ed. Elsevier Health Sciences. ISBN: 978-0-323-54387-3.

[42] Hitos, Silvia F, Arakaki, R, Solé, D, Weckx, LLM. 2013. "Oral breathing and speech disorders in children." *J Pediatr.* 89(4):361-65. https://doi.org/10.1016/j.jped.2012.12.007.

[43] Carini, Francesco, Mazzola, M, Fici, C, Messina, SPM, Damiani, P, Tomasello, G. 2017 "Posture and posturology, anatomical and

physiological profiles: overview and current state of art." *Acta Biomed.* 88(1):11-16. https://doi.org/10.23750/abm.v88i1.5309

[44] Ludwig, Oliver, Mazet, C, Mazet, D, Hammes, A, Schimitt, E. 2016. "Changes in habitual and active sagittal posture in children and adolescents with and without visual input – implications for diagnostic analysis of posture." *J Clin Diagn Res.* 10(2):SC14-7. https://doi.org/10.7860/JCDR/2016/16647.7283

[45] Scoppa, Fabio, Capra, R, Gallamini, M, Shiffer, R. 2013. "Clinical stabilometry standardization: basic definitions-acquisition interval-sampling frequency." *Gait Posture* 37(2):290-2. https://doi.org/10.1016/j.gaitpost.2012.07.009.

[46] Fensterseifer, Giovana S, Carpes, O, Weckx, LL, Martha, VF. 2013. "Mouth breathing in children with learning disorders." *Braz J Otorhinolaryngol.* 79(5):620-4. https://doi.org/10.5935/1808-8694.20130111.

[47] Hwanga, Hyeon S, Lee, KM, Uhm, GS, Cho, JH, McNamara, JA Jr. 2013. "Use of reference ear plug to improve accuracy of lateral cephalograms generated from cone-beam computed tomography scans." *Korean J Orthod.* 34(2):54-61. http://dx.doi.org/10.4041/kjod.2013.43.2.54.

[48] Vilella, Beatriz de S, Vilella, O de V, Koch, HA. 2006. "Growth of the nasopharynx and adenoidal development in Brazilian subjects." *Braz Oral Res.* 20(1):70-5. http://dx.doi.org/10.1590/S1806-83242006000100013.

[49] Pownell, Patrick, H, Minoli, JJ, Rohrich, RJ. 1997. "Diagnostic nasal endoscopy." *Plast Reconstr Surg.* 99(5):1451-8. https://doi.org/10.1097/00006534-199704001-00042.

[50] Kirk, Valerie G, Batuyong, ED, Bohn, SG. 2006. Transcutaneous carbon dioxide monitoring and capnography during pediatric polysomnography. *Sleep.* 29(12):1601-8. https://doi.org/10.1093/sleep/29.12.1601. https://doi.org/10.1093/sleep/29.12.1601.

[51] Barış, Hatice E, Gökdemir, Y, Eralp, EE, İkizoğlu, NB, Karakoç, F, Karadağ, B, Ersu, R. 2017. "Clinical and polysomnographic features of children evaluated with polysomnography in pediatric sleep

laboratory." *Türk Pediatri Arş.* 1,52(1):23-29. http://doi.org/10.5152/TurkPediatriArs.2017.4218. eCollection 2017 Mar.

[52] Tapia, Ignacio E, Karamessinis, L, Bandla, P, Huang, J, Kelly, A, Pepe, M, Schultz, B, Gallagher, P, Brooks, LJ, Marcus, C. 2008. "Polysomnographic values in children undergoing puberty: pediatric vs. adult respiratory rules in adolescents." *Sleep.* 31(12):1737-44. https://doi.org/10.1093/sleep/31.12.1737.

[53] Mitchell, RB, Pereira, KD, Friedman, NR. 2006. Sleep-disordered breathing in children: survey of current practice." *Laryngoscope.* 116(6):956-8. https://doi.org/10.1097/01.MLG.0000216413.22408. FD.

[54] Souki, Marcelo Q, Souki, BQ, Franco, LP, Becker, HMG, Araujo, EA. 2012. "Reliability of subjective, linear, ratio and area cephalometric measurements in assessing adenoid hypertrophy among different age groups." *Angle Orthod.* 82(6):1001–7. https://doi.org/10.2319/010612-13.1.

[55] McNamara, James A Jr. 1981. "Influence of respiratory pattern on craniofacial growth." *Angle Orthod.* 51(4):269-300. https://www.angle.org/doi/pdf/10.1043/0003-3219%281981%29051%3C0269%3AIORPOC%3E2.0.CO%3B2

[56] McNamara, James A Jr. 1984. "A method of cephalometric evaluation." *Am J Orthod.* 86(6):449–69. https://doi.org/10.1016/S0002-9416(84)90352-X.

[57] Faria, Patrícia TM, Ruellas, ACO, Matsumoto, MAN, Anselmo-Lima, WT, Pereira, FC. 2002. "Dentofacial morphology of mouth breathing children." *Braz Dent J.* 13(2):129-32. http://dx.doi.org/10.1590/S0103-64402002000200010.

[58] Major, Michael P, Flores-Mir, C, Major, PW. 2006. "Assessment of lateral cephalometric diagnosis of adenoid hypertrophy and posterior upper airway obstruction: a systematic review." *Am J Orthod Dentofacial Orthop.* 130(6):700-8. https://doi.org/10.1016/j.ajodo.2005.05.050.

[59] Pirila-Parkkinen, Kirsi, Lopponen, H, Nieminen, P, Tolonen, U, Paakko, E, Pirttiniemi, P. 2011. "Validity of upper airway assessment

in children: a clinical, cephalometric, and MRI study." *Angle Orthodont.* 81(3):433-39. https://doi.org/10.2319/063010-362.1.

[60] Ballista, Paula R. 2016. *"Alterações da morfologia craniofacial e da via aérea superior em crianças com obstrução na nasofaringe."* (Craniofacial and upper airway morphology changes in children with nasopharyngeal obstruction) 81p. MS diss. Universidade Federal do Espírito Santo, Vitória. http://repositorio.ufes.br/bitstream/10/8087/1/tese_10049_Disserta%C3%A7%C3%A3o%20Mestrado%20-%20Paula%20Ramos%20Ballista%20%281%29%20%281%29.pdf

[61] Praud, Jean-Paul and Dominique Dorion. 2008. "Obstructive sleep disordered breathing in children: beyond adenotonsillectomy." *Pediatr Pulmonol.* 43(9):837-43. https://doi.org/10.1002/ppul.20888.

[62] Puri, Prem. 2016, "The 29th international symposium on paediatric surgical research." *Pediatr Surg Int.* 32(12):1093 https://doi.org/10.1007/s00383-016-3981-3

[63] Camelo-Nunes, Inês C and Dirceu Solé. 2010. "Allergic rhinitis: indicators of quality of life." *J Bras Pneumol.* 36(1):124-33. http://dx.doi.org/10.1590/S1806-37132010000100017.

[64] Huynh, Nelly T, Desplats, E, Almeida, FR. 2016. "Orthodontics treatments for managing obstructive sleep apnea syndrome in children: a systematic review and meta-analysis." *Sleep Medicine Reviews.* 25:84-94. https://doi.org/10.1016/j.smrv.2015.02.002.

[65] Camacho, Macario, Chang, ET, Song, SA, Abdullatif, J, Zaghi, S, Pirelli, P, Certal, V, Guilleminault, C. 2017. "Rapid maxillary expansion for pediatric obstructive sleep apnea: a systematic review and meta-analysis." *Laryngoscope.* 127(7):1712-19. https://doi.org/10.1002/lary.26352.

[66] Wells, Andrew, P, Sarver, DM, Proffit, WR. 2006. "Long-term efficacy of reverse pull headgear therapy." *Angle Orthod.* 76(6):915-22. https://doi.org/10.2319/091605-328.

[67] Nguyen, Tung, De Clerck, H, Wilson, M, Golden, B. 2015. "Effect of Class III bone anchor treatment on airway." *Angle Orthod.* 85(4):591-6. https://doi.org/10.2319/041614-282.1.

[68] Lee, Ji-Won, Park, KH, Kim, SH, Park, YG, Kim, SJ. 2011." Correlation between skeletal changes by maxillary protraction and upper airway dimensions." *Angle Orthod.* 81(3):426-32. https://doi.org/10.2319/082610-499.1.

[69] Danaei, Shahla, M, Ajami, S, Etemadi, H, Azadeh, N. 2018. "Assessment of the effect of maxillary protraction appliance on pharyngeal airway dimensions in relation to changes in tongue posture." *Dent Res J.* (Isfahan)15(3):208-14.

[70] Schütz, Teresa Cristina B, Dominguez, GC, Hallinan, MP, Cunha, TC, Tufik, S. 2011. "Class II correction improves nocturnal breathing in adolescents." *Angle Orthod.* 81(2):222-8. https://doi.org/10.2319/052710-233.1.

[71] Iwasaki, Tomonori, Takemoto, Y, Inada, E, Sato, H, Saitoh, I, Kakuno, E, Kanomi, R, Yamasaki, Y. 2014. "Three-dimensional cone-beam computed tomography analysis of enlargement of the pharyngeal airway by the Herbst appliance." *Am J Orthod Dentofacial Orthop.* 146(6):776-85. https://doi.org/10.1016/j.ajodo.2014.08.017.

[72] Iwasaki, Tomonori, Sato H, Suga H, Minami A, Yamamoto Y, Takemoto Y, Inada E, Saitoh, I, Kakuno, E, Kanomi, R, Yamasaki, Y. 2017. "Herbst appliance effects on pharyngeal airway ventilation evaluated using computational fluid dynamics." *Angle Orthod.* 87(3):397-403. https://doi.org/10.2319/080616-603.1.

[73] Itzhaki, Sarah, Dorchin, H, Clark, G, Lavie, L, Lavie, P, Pillar, G. 2007. "The effects of 1-year treatment with a Herbst mandibular advancement splint on obstructive sleep apnea, oxidative stress, and endothelial function." *Chest.* 131(3):740-749. https://doi.org/10.1378/chest.06-0965.

[74] Serra-Torres, Sara, Bellot-Arcís, C, Montiel-Company, JM, Marco-Algarra, J, Almerich-Silla, JM. 2016 "Effectiveness of mandibular advancement appliances in treating obstructive sleep apnea syndrome: a systematic review." *Laryngoscope.* 126(2):507-14. https://doi.org/10.1002/lary.25505.

[75] Pancherz, Hans, Bjerklin, K, Lindskog-Stokland, B, Hansen, K. 2014. "Thirty-two-year follow-up study of Herbst therapy: a biometric dental

cast analysis." *Am J Orthod Dentofacial Orthop.* 145(1):15-27. http://dx.doi.org/10.1016/j.ajodo.2013.09.012.

[76] Pancherz, Hans, Salé, H, Bjerklin, K. 2015. "Signs and symptoms of TMJ disorders in adults after adolescent Herbst therapy: a 6-year and 32-year radiographic and clinical follow-up study." *Angle Orthod.* 85(5):735-42. https://doi.org/10.2319/072914-530.1.

[77] Lee, Seo-Young, Guilleminault, C, Chiu, HY, Sullivan, SS. 2015. "Mouth breathing, "nasal disuse," and pediatric sleep-disordered breathing." *Sleep and Breathing.* 19(4):1257-64. https://doi.org/10.1007/s11325-015-1154-6

[78] Rosario Jose L. 2017. "Understanding muscular chains – a review for clinical application of chain stretching exercises aimed to correct posture." *EC Orthopaedics.* 5(6): 209-234.

[79] Vanti Carla, Generali A, Ferrari S, Nava T, Tosarelli D, Pillastrini P. 2007. "General postural rehabilitation in musculoskeletal diseases: scientific evidence and clinical indications." *Reumatismo.* 59(3):192-201.

[80] Capdevila, Oscar S, Kheirandish-Gozal L, Dayyat E, Gozal D. 2008. "Pediatric obstructive sleep apnea: complications, management, and long-term outcomes." *Proc Am Thorac Soc.* 15,5(2):274-82. DOI: https://doi.org/10.1513/pats.200708-138MG

[81] Kuhle, Stefan, Urschitz, MS, Eitner, S, Poets, CF. 2009. "Interventions for obstructive sleep apnea in children: a systematic review." *Sleep Med Rev.* 13(2):123-31. http://doi.org/10.1016/j.smrv.2008.07.006. Epub 2008 Dec 6

[82] Andrade, Rafaela GS, Piccin, VS, Nascimento, JA, Viana, FML, Genta, PR, Lorenzi-Filho, G. 2014. "Impact of the type of mask on the effectiveness of and adherence to continuous positive airway pressure treatment for obstructive sleep apnea." *J Bras Pneumol.* 40(6):658-668. http://dx.doi.org/10.1590/S1806-37132014000600010.

BIOGRAPHICAL SKETCHES

Maria Christina Thomé Pacheco, PhD

Affiliation: Department of Dental Clinic, Federal University of Espírito Santo. Vitória – ES, Brazil.

Education: PhD in Orthodontics; Dental Radiology expert.

Research and Professional Experience: Professor of Orthodontics and Dental Radiology. Main research areas: Dentistry, Orthodontics, Radiology and Imaging, with emphasis on facial cranium growth and development, facial orthopedics, preventive, interceptive and corrective orthodontics; dental materials, biomechanics, obstructive sleep breathing disorders, radiographic and tomographic images.

Professional Appointments: Full Professor of the Department of Dental Clinic/Federal University of Espírito Santo. Postdoctoral fellow (2008 – 2009) Department of Biomaterials/Military Engineering Institute, Rio de Janeiro – Brazil.

Honors: President of the Society of Orthodontists of Espírito Santo - 1996-1998. President of the Association of Postgraduates in Orthodontics of Federal University of Rio de Janeiro - 2000-2002. President of the XII Meeting of Postgraduates in Orthodontics of Federal University of Rio de Janeiro – 2002.

Publications from the Last 3 Years:
1. de Araújo MTM, Pacheco MCT. (2018). *Distúrbios respiratórios na infância: da respiração oral à apneia obstrutiva do sono* [*Respiratory disorders in childhood: from mouth breathing to obstructive sleep apnea*]. Ed 1. Vitória, ES, Brazil 1: 1-96. UFES.
2. Brandão RCB, Silva CA, Pacheco MCT. (2017) Abordagem da Microestética na Ortodontia [Microesthesia Approach in

Orthodontics]. In: *Ortodontia – Estado atual da arte – diagnostico, planejamento e tratamento* [Orthodontics - State of the art - diagnosis, planning and treatment]. Ed 1, Nova Odessa, SP, Brazil 1: 232-257. Napoleão.

3. Ribeiro AF, Morosini LM, Finck NS, Pacheco MCT, Araújo MTM. (2016) Associação entre as adaptações da articulação temporomandibular e a qualidade de vida de escolares respiradores bucais [Association between adaptations of the temporomandibular joint and the quality of life of school mouth breathers]. *Fisioterapia Brasil*, 17: 321-334.

Fabiana Vasconcelos Campos, PhD

Affiliation: Department of Physiological Sciences, Federal University of Espírito Santo. Avenida Maruípe, 1468, Vitória – ES, Brazil 29040-090.

Education: PhD in Biochemistry and Immunology.

Research and Professional Experience: Main research areas: Biophysics of voltage-gated ion channels; pharmacology of animal toxins and venoms; protein biochemistry; cell and molecular biology; English to Portuguese professional translation.

Professional Appointments: Postdoctoral fellow (2016 – present day) at the Department of Physiological Sciences/Federal University of Espírito Santo – Brazil. Research Technician (2012 - 2013) at the Cell Biology and Biophysics Department/European Molecular Biology Laboratory – Germany. Postdoctoral fellow (2009-2011) at the Department of Biological and Environmental Sciences/University of Jyvä skylä – Finland. Postdoctoral fellow (2006 - 2008) at the Department of Molecular Pediatric Sciences/University of Chicago – USA. Visiting PhD student (January 2005–November 2005) at the Department of Physiology/University of California Los Angeles – USA.

Honors: International Travel Grant from the American Biophysical Society 2002.

Publications from the Last 3 Years:
1. Pimenta FS, Tose H, Waichert Jr. E, Da Cunha MRH, Campos FV et al. (2019) *Lipids in Health and Disease.* 18(1):44.
2. Borges YG, Cipriano LHC, Aires R, Zovico PVC, Campos FV, de Araújo MTM et al. (2019) *Sleep and Breathing.* 23:1-9.
3. Malacarne PF, Menezes TN, Martins CW, Naumann GB, Gomes HL, Pires RGW, Figueiredo SG, Campos FV. (2018) *Toxicon.* 150: 220-27.
4. Borges MH, Andrich F, Lemos PH, Soares TG, Menezes TN, Campos FV et al. (2018) *Journal of Proteomics.* 187: 200-11.
5. Campos FV et al. (2016) *Journal of Venomous Animals and Toxins including Tropical Diseases.* 22: 1-9.

Maria Teresa Martins de Araújo, PhD

Affiliation: Department of Physiological Sciences, Federal University of Espírito Santo. Avenida Maruípe, 1468, Vitória – ES, Brazil 29040-090.

Education: PhD in Physiological Sciences.

Research and Professional Experience: Professor of Physiology. Main research areas: physiology, with emphasis on cardiorespiratory physiology. Specializes on the following subjects: mouth breathing, cardiorespiratory disorders, musculoskeletal, cognitive and dental changes resulting from sleep disorders, especially in Obstructive Sleep Apnea.

Professional Appointments: Professor of the Department of Physiological Sciences and coordinator of the Laboratory of Sleep Respiratory Disorders at the Federal University of Espírito Santo.

Publications from the Last 3 Years:

1. Borges YG, Cipriano LHC, Aires R, Zovico PVC, Campos FV, de Araújo MTM, Gouvea SA. (2019) *Sleep and Breathing.* 23: 1-9.
2. de Araújo MTM, Pacheco MCT. (2018). *Distúrbios respiratórios na infância: da respiração oral à apneia obstrutiva do sono sono* [*Respiratory disorders in childhood: from mouth breathing to obstructive sleep apnea*] . Ed 1. Vitória, ES, Brazil. 1: 1-96. UFES.
3. Gouvea AS, Oliveira KG, Araújo MTM, Silva FB, Thebit MM, Silva AVB. (2017) Hypertensive Retinopathy: Pathophysicology and Clinical Management. In: *Arterioles Dynamic Structure, Function and Clinical Analisys.* Ed 1. New York. Chapter 3, 1: 77-104. Nova Biomedical.
4. Ribeiro AF, Morosini LM, Finck NS, Pacheco MCT, Araújo MTM. (2016) Associação entre as adaptações da articulação temporomandibular e a qualidade de vida de escolares respiradores bucais [Association between adaptations of the temporomandibular joint and the quality of life of school mouth breathers]. *Fisioterapia Brasil*, 17: 321-334.

INDEX

A

actigraphy, vii, viii, 1, 2, 7, 8, 9, 10, 11, 12, 21, 23, 24, 26, 27, 28, 29, 30
adenoidectomy, 142
adenoids, 43
adeno-tonsillar hypertrophy, 128
adolescents, vii, viii, 1, 11, 14, 16, 17, 20, 22, 24, 27, 29, 31, 32, 33, 35, 38, 40, 44, 47, 48, 49, 64, 65, 67, 68, 70, 71, 72, 74, 75, 81, 86, 88, 90, 92, 97, 102, 106, 108, 110, 111, 160, 161, 163
anterior facial height, 119
anterior open bite, 119, 121, 124, 132, 143, 146
anxiety disorder, 57, 101, 102, 104, 108, 110, 111, 114
assessment, v, viii, 1, 2, 4, 5, 6, 9, 10, 11, 13, 14, 16, 18, 21, 22, 23, 25, 27, 28, 30, 61, 65, 67, 68, 75, 91, 110, 131, 132, 133, 135, 138, 158, 159, 161, 163
assessment tools, 16, 22, 23
asthma, 44, 66, 129
attention deficit, 32, 62, 63, 80, 88, 102, 103, 106, 109, 127
Attention Deficit Hyperactivity Disorder, (ADHD), 32, 34, 39, 43, 45, 46, 59, 60, 62, 63, 111, 112
autism, 34, 87, 88, 110

B

behavior, ix, 17, 24, 29, 39, 53, 57, 60, 63, 77, 80, 84, 94, 97, 100, 103, 105, 106, 112, 121, 128, 134
behavior therapy, 29
behavioral change, 127
behavioral disorders, 8, 61, 103
behavioral problems, vii, x, 8, 57, 80, 83, 88, 90, 100, 103, 110
behaviors, 15, 16, 20, 37, 39, 58, 73, 85, 88, 90, 91, 92
body posture, xi, 116, 121, 124, 150
bone growth, 121, 138
breathing, vii, x, xi, 4, 18, 21, 25, 27, 29, 33, 40, 43, 45, 52, 66, 69, 71, 72, 75, 76, 82, 91, 93, 105, 107, 110, 116, 117, 118, 119, 120, 121, 122, 123, 124, 125, 126, 127, 129, 131, 132, 133, 134, 135, 136, 140, 141, 142, 143, 146, 150, 151, 152,

154, 155, 156, 157, 158, 159, 160, 161, 162, 163, 164, 165, 167
breathing disorders, vii, x, xi, 116, 118, 119, 129, 135, 140, 142, 143, 151, 152, 155, 158, 165
Brodsky degrees, 130

C

caffeine, 48, 49, 52, 59
capnography, xi, 116, 136, 160
Cavum radiography, 135
cervical vertebrae maturation, 148
Child Behavior Checklist, 24, 105
circadian rhythm sleep-wake disorder - delayed sleep phase type, 32, 46, 61, 62, 63
circadian rhythms, 24, 37, 106
clinical management, 141, 168
clinical presentation, 32, 34, 61, 112
cognitive flexibility, ix, 80, 88, 92
cognitive function, ix, 80, 96
cognitive performance, 85, 92, 113
constricted palate, 121
continuous positive airway pressure (CPAP), 149, 152, 164
craniofacial alterations, x, 116, 120, 128, 150
crossbite, 119, 121, 147, 148

D

deleterious oral habits, xi, 116, 118, 143, 144
depression, ix, 33, 34, 40, 42, 43, 50, 60, 66, 80, 91, 100, 101, 102, 104, 105, 109, 110, 111, 112, 113
depressive symptomatology, 103
depressive symptoms, 67, 104
detection, viii, 31, 32, 61, 134, 150
developmental change, 97, 110

diagnostic criteria, ix, 32, 33, 45, 67, 74, 100, 101, 136

E

emotions, 54, 100, 102
excessive daytime sleepiness, 4, 18, 37, 38, 39, 40, 43, 45, 47, 57, 60, 66, 76, 100, 105, 108, 109, 126
externalizing behavior, 45, 60, 106
externalizing disorders, ix, 100, 101, 102
extraoral device, 147
eye movement, ix, 3, 52, 80, 82

F

facial and dental skeletal deformities, 121
facial asymmetry, 125
facial axes, 144
facial expression, 82
facial mask, 147, 148
family history, 47, 52, 59, 129
forward head posture, 124
frontal lobe, 78

G

generalized anxiety disorder, x, 100, 101, 102
genetic factors, 42, 123
genetic predisposition, 52
genetic syndromes, 128
genetics, 85, 148
gestational age, 83
glomerulus, 91
gray matter, 83, 86, 87, 91, 97
growth, 45, 82, 87, 118, 119, 120, 121, 123, 124, 131, 134, 135, 139, 142, 143, 147, 148, 154, 161, 165
growth spurt, 144, 148

H

health, ix, 61, 80, 82, 88, 89, 90, 94, 95, 153
hyoid, 118, 124, 139
hyperactivity, ix, 8, 32, 39, 45, 56, 60, 62, 63, 76, 77, 80, 88, 102, 103, 106, 109, 110, 125, 127, 128, 134, 136
hypercapnia, 126, 128
hypersomnia, 8, 64, 65, 68
hypersomnolence disorder, 22, 32, 37, 38, 40, 42, 61, 62, 63
hypertension, ix, 80, 128, 135
hypertrophy, 119, 120, 124, 125, 127, 129, 131, 135, 136, 138, 142, 161
hypertrophy of the adenoid, 120, 127
hypertrophy of the palatine tonsils, 135
hypertrophy of the tonsils, 119
hypnagogic hallucinations, 41, 43
hypoxemia, 128
hypoxia, 128, 158, 159

I

impulsive, 88
impulsivity, 45, 60, 89, 90, 97, 106
inferior turbinate hypertrophy, 120, 124
insomnia, 4, 8, 12, 13, 15, 22, 25, 26, 27, 29, 32, 33, 34, 35, 36, 46, 49, 56, 57, 61, 63, 65, 66, 69, 70, 74, 77, 89, 101, 106, 110, 111, 112
insomnia disorder, 33, 62, 63
intellectual disabilities, 34, 83
intelligence quotient, 83
international classification of sleep disorders – ICSD-3, 136
intraoral device, 147, 148
irritability, 37, 102

K

kyphosis, 124

L

laryngopharynx, 149
larynx, 118
lateral cephalometric radiography (LCR), 129, 135, 137, 138, 139, 148
learning difficulties, 80, 125
learning disabilities, 129
learning impairment, 127
learning skills, 83
lip sealing, 121, 124, 131, 132, 143, 146
long face, 122, 123
loss of consciousness, 41
lower lip, 121, 131
lower third of the face, 121
lumbar spine, 133
lung function, 140
lymphoid tissue, 127, 142

M

Mallampati score, 124, 129, 130
malocclusion(s), 119, 121, 139, 143, 145, 146, 147, 149
mandible, 119, 121, 124, 125, 131, 132, 139, 143, 144, 148
mandibular retrusion, 135, 144, 148, 149
maxilla, 117, 118, 119, 121, 122, 131, 144, 146, 147, 148, 149
maxillary constriction, 124, 145
maxillary protraction, 143, 144, 147, 163
maxillary retrusion, 147, 148
medication, 37, 63, 129, 142
medicine, 67, 110, 129
melatonin, 48, 84
memory, 54, 83, 85, 88, 90, 92, 97, 128, 134

memory formation, 86, 88
memory performance, 97
mental disorder, 22, 32, 40, 54, 57, 64, 71
mental health, 2, 32, 50, 60, 80, 92, 97
meta-analysis, 26, 27, 29, 76, 109, 144, 146, 162
metabolic disorders, 39
metabolic syndrome, 80
metabolism, 80, 84, 87
middle third of the face, 144, 147
midpalatal suture, 144, 145
migraine headache, 59
migraines, 42, 52
morphology, ix, 66, 80, 86, 91, 131, 134, 155, 161, 162
motor activity, 39, 43, 58
mouth breather, 120, 121, 124, 125, 133, 151, 152, 156, 166, 168
mouth breathing, vi, vii, x, xi, 45, 91, 115, 116, 118, 119, 120, 121, 122, 123, 124, 125, 126, 127, 129, 132, 133, 134, 140, 141, 142, 143, 150, 152, 154, 155, 156, 157, 158, 161, 165, 167, 168
muscles, 60, 82, 118, 119, 121, 124, 125, 128, 140, 143, 150, 152
musculoskeletal, 121, 164, 167
myelin, 86, 95

N

narcolepsy, 4, 17, 22, 32, 40, 41, 42, 43, 46, 61, 62, 63, 64, 65, 69, 70, 72, 73, 76, 77, 95
nasal breathing, x, xi, 116, 117, 118, 122, 123, 150
nasal septum deviation, 124
nasofibroscopy, 129, 136
network analysis, 100, 103
neural development, 94
neural function, 88
neural networks, 86, 89, 92

neurodevelopmental disorders, 34, 89, 93
neurogenesis, 90
neurological disease, 128, 135
neuronal apoptosis, 128
night terrors, 109
nightmare disorder, 4, 22, 32, 54, 55, 57, 61, 62, 63
nightmares, 11, 15, 54, 55, 56, 57, 71, 75, 76, 100, 101, 113
non-nutritive sucking, 123
non-rapid eye movement sleep arousal disorder (Non-REM (NREM)), 32, 50, 61

O

obesity, ix, 42, 44, 66, 73, 77, 80, 134, 153, 157
obstructive sleep apnea (OSA), vii, x, xi, 4, 17, 22, 26, 32, 42, 43, 44, 61, 62, 63, 66, 67, 72, 73, 74, 76, 115, 116, 118, 126, 127, 128, 129, 134, 136, 137, 138, 140, 141, 142, 143, 146, 148, 152, 153, 154, 156, 158, 159, 162, 163, 164, 165, 167, 168
obstructive sleep apnea hypopnea (OSAH), 22, 32, 43, 44, 45, 46, 52, 60, 61, 62, 63
occlusion, 133, 144, 149
onset latency, 11, 12, 104
oral cavity, 118, 129
oropharynx, 120, 139, 149
orthodontic and facial orthopedic treatments, 142, 143
orthodontic treatment, 142
orthopedic mandibular advancement, 144
otitis media, 127
otolaryngologist, 142
oxyhemoglobin, 136, 153

Index

P

palate, x, 116, 117, 118, 121, 133, 135, 138, 144, 146, 150
parasomnias, 4, 13, 40, 45, 50, 54, 60, 62, 63, 68, 70, 72, 74, 76, 78, 95, 103, 105, 107, 110, 111, 112
patency of the UA, 124
pathology, 10, 21, 32, 71
pathophysiology, 67, 106
pathways, 83, 87, 104, 112
pediatric obstructive sleep apnea (OSA)/pediatric OSA, vi, x, 44, 64, 115, 116, 126, 128, 136, 137, 139, 140, 141, 144, 146, 147, 150, 152, 154, 155, 164
pharynx, 118, 153
polysomnography, vii, viii, xi, 1, 2, 21, 23, 24, 25, 26, 29, 30, 41, 44, 46, 65, 116, 129, 136, 137, 139, 153, 160
positive airway pressure (PAP), 140, 152, 153, 154
posterior crossbite, 121, 124, 132, 144, 145
preschool children, 55, 83, 87
protrusion, 119, 124, 148, 150
psychiatric disorders, 103, 109
psychiatry, 55, 109, 113
psychological distress, 42, 75
psychological problems, ix, 80
psychology, 109, 112, 114
psychometric properties, 12, 13, 19, 21, 23, 112
psychopathology, 2, 22, 69, 101, 108
psychosocial factors, 47, 85
pubertal growth spurt, 144, 148
puberty, 34, 42, 62, 83, 89, 124, 148, 161
pulmonary hypertension, 128

Q

quality of life, 42, 88, 141, 142, 153, 157, 162

questionnaires, vii, viii, 1, 2, 15, 16, 18, 19, 20, 21, 29

R

rapid eye movement sleep, 32, 61, 70
rapid maxillary expansion (RME), 143, 144, 145, 155
respiratory arrests, 127
respiratory effort-related arousal (RERA), 118, 126, 137
respiratory problems, 157
restless legs syndrome (RLS), 4, 13, 17, 22, 32, 36, 49, 52, 58, 59, 60, 61, 62, 63, 64, 65, 73, 74, 77, 78

S

schizophrenia, 43, 57, 77
school performance, 49, 67, 89, 92, 127, 129, 134
serotonin, 104, 111
sleep apnea, 13, 24, 43, 60, 62, 63, 66, 67, 87, 91, 110, 126, 158
sleep deprivation, 43, 47, 52, 87, 89, 90, 113
sleep diaries, vii, viii, 1, 2, 8, 9, 11, 12, 13, 14, 21, 28, 29
sleep disorders, v, vii, viii, 1, 2, 5, 8, 17, 18, 19, 21, 22, 24, 27, 29, 30, 31, 32, 33, 40, 42, 43, 46, 61, 62, 63, 65, 66, 67, 68, 70, 72, 74, 75, 81, 86, 87, 88, 90, 92, 93, 94, 111, 112, 136, 137, 157, 159, 167
sleep disturbances, vii, viii, ix, x, 18, 20, 25, 32, 52, 68, 79, 87, 88, 90, 91, 94, 95, 99, 100, 103, 106, 107, 114
sleep fragmentation, 107, 126
sleep habits, 15, 20, 49
sleep hygiene, 49, 62, 63, 66, 141
sleep latency, 24, 134
sleep medicine, 10, 22, 28, 29, 66, 74, 112, 156

sleep paralysis, 41
sleep spindle, 82, 86, 93
sleep terrors, 50, 51, 52, 57, 100, 110
sleep walking, 50
sleep-disordered breathing, xi, 25, 29, 33, 72, 91, 116, 126, 154, 155, 157, 158, 159, 164
sleep-related breathing disorders, x, 75, 116, 129, 140
smoke exposure, 69
smoking, 89
snoring, 3, 15, 16, 18, 40, 43, 45, 46, 63, 88, 91, 93, 118, 126, 127, 134, 136, 144, 153
stomatognathic system, x, 116, 118, 140, 150
symptoms, vii, x, xi, 20, 32, 33, 36, 37, 38, 40, 42, 43, 44, 45, 46, 48, 49, 59, 60, 61, 66, 67, 71, 76, 91, 100, 101, 103, 105, 106, 108, 110, 113, 116, 127, 128, 136, 141, 142, 155, 164
synaptic plasticity, 87, 89, 90

T

teeth, x, 107, 116, 118, 120, 121, 123, 131, 143, 144, 145, 147, 148, 150
temporomandibular joint (TMJ), 125, 157, 164, 166, 168
therapy, 114, 140, 142, 150, 151, 152, 162, 163, 164
tongue, 117, 118, 119, 121, 122, 123, 124, 128, 130, 132, 133, 143, 146, 150, 163

tongue interposition, 119, 143
tonsillectomy, 142
tonsillitis, 142
tonsils, 43, 119, 120, 124, 127, 130, 133, 135, 139, 141, 142, 146, 159

U

UA obstructions, 119, 138
upper airway (UA), x, xi, 44, 115, 116, 117, 118, 119, 120, 123, 126, 127, 129, 132, 135, 136, 137, 138, 139, 140, 142, 143, 144, 146, 147, 153, 154, 157, 161, 162, 163
upper respiratory tract, 127, 134
uvula, 129, 150

V

vertical and anteroposterior, 144, 146

W

waking, ix, 28, 40, 48, 49, 99, 100, 103, 105, 106, 107, 113, 125

Y

youth populations, 34, 42